W9-BXB-755

BY THE SAME AUTHOR

The Farmers' Market Cookbook

real food

WHAT TO EAT AND WHY

NINA PLANCK

BLOOMSBURY

Copyright © 2006 by Nina Planck

All rights reserved. No part of this book may be used
or reproduced in any manner whatsoever without written permission from the publisher
except in the case of brief quotations embodied in critical articles or
reviews. For information address
Bloomsbury Publishing, 175 Fifth Avenue, New York, NY 10010.

Published by Bloomsbury Publishing, New York and London
Distributed to the trade by Holtzbrinck Publishers

The ideas and suggestions in this book are not
intended to replace the services of a health professional.
The reader is advised to take professional advice before
making significant changes in diet.

All papers used by Bloomsbury Publishing are natural, recyclable
products made from wood grown in well-managed forests. The
manufacturing processes conform to the environmental regulations
of the country of origin.

Library of Congress Cataloging-in-Publication Data

Planck, Nina, 1971–
Real food: what to eat and why / Nina Planck.
p. cm.
Includes bibliographical references.
ISBN-13: 978-1-59691-144-4 (hardcover)
ISBN-10: 1-59691-144-1 (hardcover)
1. Nutrition—United States. 2. Diet—United States. I. Title.

TX360.U6P63 2006
613.20973—dc22
2005033624

First U.S. Edition 2006

5 7 9 10 8 6 4

Typeset by Palimpsest Book Production Ltd, Polmont, Stirlingshire
Printed in the United States of America by
Quebecor World Fairfield

Contents

1

I Grow Up on Real Food, Lose My Way, and Come Home Again

First I Explain What Real Food Is

WHEN I WAS GROWING UP on a vegetable farm in Loudoun County, Virginia, we ate what I now think of as *real food*. Just about everything at our table was local, seasonal, and homemade. Eating our own fresh vegetables certainly made me proud; they tasted better than the supermarket vegetables other people ate. But I regarded homemade granola, whole wheat bread, and chicken livers—not to mention the notable lack of store-bought processed foods in brightly colored boxes in our kitchen—as uncool. Today, my embarrassment over the simple American meals we ate is long gone, and I regard the food I grew up on as the very best. It's true that in certain quarters these days, sautéed chicken livers *are* fashionable, but I don't care about that; I prefer real food because it's delicious and it's healthy.

What is *real food*? My rough definition has two parts. First, real foods are *old*. These are foods we've been eating for a long time—in the case of meat, fish, and eggs, for millions of years. Some real foods, such as butter, are more recent. It's not absolutely clear when regular dairy farming began, but we've been eating butterfat for at least ten thousand years, perhaps as many as forty thousand. By contrast, margarine—hydrogenated vegetable oil made solid and dyed yellow to resemble traditional butter—is a modern invention, merely a century old. Margarine is not a real food.

Consider the soybean. Asians have been eating foods made from fermented soybeans, such as miso, tofu, and soy sauce, for about five thousand years. Without fermentation, the soybean isn't ideal for human consumption. But most of the modern soy products Americans eat are not traditional soy foods. The main ingredient in modern soy foods and many processed foods, such as low-carbohydrate snack bars, is "isolated soy protein," a by-product of the industrial soybean oil industry. This unfermented, defatted soy protein is not real food.

Second, real foods are *traditional.* To me, *traditional* means "the way we used to eat them." That means different things for different ingredients: fruits and vegetables are best when they're local and seasonal; grains should be whole; fats and oils unrefined. From the farm to the factory to the kitchen, real food is produced and prepared the old-fashioned way—but not out of mere nostalgia. In each of these examples of real food, the traditional method of farming, processing, preparing, and cooking *enhances* nutrition and flavor, while the industrial method diminishes both.

- Real *beef* is raised on grass (not soybeans) and aged properly.
- Real *milk* is grass-fed, raw, and unhomogenized, with the cream on top.
- Real *eggs* come from hens that eat grass, grubs, and bugs—not "vegetarian" hens.
- Real *lard* is never hydrogenated, as industrial lard is.
- Real *olive oil* is cold-pressed, leaving vitamin E and antioxidants intact.
- Real *tofu* is made from fermented soybeans, which are more digestible.

- Real *bread* is made with yeast and allowed to rise, a form of fermentation.
- Real *grits* are stone-ground from whole corn and soaked with soda before cooking.

Industrial food is the opposite of real food. Real food is old and traditional, while industrial food is recent and synthetic. The impersonation of real food by industrial food, by the way, is neither accidental nor hidden. Industrial food like margarine is *intended* to be a replica of a traditional food—butter. Real food is fundamentally conservative; it doesn't change, while industrial food, by contrast, is under great pressure to be novel. The food industry is highly competitive and relentlessly innovative, producing thousands of new food products every year. Most of these "new" foods are merely new combinations of old ingredients dressed in a new shape (individually wrapped cheese slices instead of the traditional wheel of pressed cheese) or new packaging (whipped cream in an aerosol can). Or the new recipe has been tweaked to ride the latest food craze (cholesterol-free cheese, low-carbohydrate bagels). Real food, on the other hand, doesn't change because it doesn't have to. My morning yogurt is a masterfully simple recipe for cultured milk, passed down for thousands of years.

So that's my custom definition of *real food*: it's old, and it's traditional. To lexicographers, sticklers, and nitpickers (you know who you are), it's no doubt hopelessly imprecise and incomplete, but I hope it's clear enough for our purposes.

People everywhere love traditional foods. They're fond of a nice steak, the crispy skin of roast chicken, or mashed potatoes made with plenty of milk and butter. But they're afraid that eating these things might make them fat—or, worse, give them a heart attack. So they do as they're told by the experts: they drink skim milk and order egg white omelets. Their favorite foods become a guilty pleasure. I believe the experts are wrong; the real culprits in heart disease are not traditional foods but industrial ones, such as margarine, powdered eggs, refined corn oil, and sugar. Real food is good for you.

Does that mean you should enjoy real bacon and butter not because they're tasty but because they're actually *healthy*? In a word, yes. Some might mock this as a characteristically American case for real food—call it the Virtue Defense. Gina Mallet, an Anglo-American "food explorer" who defends real foods, including beef and raw milk cheese, in *Last Chance to Eat: The Fate of Taste in a Fast Food World*, calls the modish philosophy *healthism*—and her intent is not to flatter. As scientists began to blame the diseases of civilization on diet, Mallet writes, "a new philosophy emerged, based on the notion that death could be delayed, perhaps even cheated, if a person monitored every single piece of food she ate." I'm concerned about nutrition, but I wouldn't call myself a healthist. For one thing, living forever doesn't interest me, and for another, flavor does.

Someone else—a French chef perhaps—might take a different approach in defense of real food. Less interested in health, he might champion pleasure for its own sake. Great—I'm all for pleasure. If the sheer sensual joy of eating shirred eggs or homemade ice cream is enough for you to shed your guilt, throw away phony industrial foods, and return to eating real foods, all the better. I'll leave the nature of taste and satisfaction, guilt and pleasure to the cultural critics and moral philosophers. *This* book is about why real food is good for you.

We Become Vegetable Farmers in Virginia

MY PARENTS CHOSE TO FARM, but I didn't. My father had a doctorate in international relations from Johns Hopkins and taught political science at the State University of New York in Buffalo, where I was born in 1971. A bright young professor, he got tenure early, and he could teach anything he wanted. My mother, for her part, was at home with three young children and very happy. But they always had unconventional plans and utopian ideas: unsatisfied with our local public school in Buffalo, they started and ran a neighborhood school with other parents. They loved physical work and kept a plot in a garden outside of town.

In January 1973, our friends Tony and Mariette Newcomb came to see us in Buffalo. They brought eggs and beef they had raised on their farm in Virginia. "We were knocked out by that," my father said. That very year, Dad quit teaching and we moved south to Virginia to learn vegetable farming from the Newcombs. Committed to farming before they'd even tried it, they also bought sixty acres of farmland in Loudoun County, Virginia, for seventy-five thousand dollars they cobbled together with loans from friends and family. My sister, Hilary, was ten years old, Charles was six, and I was two. They wanted us to grow up on a farm.

Our first years farming as apprentices to the Newcombs were wonderful and strange, very different from the life of a professor's family. Mom and Dad worked all the time, and we lived simply. With no kids my age to play with, I was often lonely hanging around the farm or playing at make-believe grocery shopping at our farm stand. In many ways it was a hard life. But however sore and tired they were, my parents loved farming, and soon we moved west to our own place, in the tiny hamlet of Wheatland, Virginia. We arrived at the farm late on Christmas Eve in 1978. All our things, including a few pieces of farm equipment, were tied up in a rickety pile on the back of our green flatbed Ford. There was too much snow to drive up to the house, and there was no driveway anyway, so we parked at the edge of the property and walked a quarter of a mile.

The old tenant house had little charm. The kitchen floor was covered with a dirty mustard carpet. Under that was linoleum; under that, plywood, hiding yellow pine floorboards. The sink drained through the kitchen wall into the backyard. We heated the house and water for baths with wood fires. But my parents are relentlessly cheerful and practical, and over the years we fixed up the house, scrubbing, scraping, and painting, with the simple faith that natural materials, such as wood floors, are beautiful no matter how modest or worn.

In the spring of 1979, we became farmers. While other kids played soccer and went to the beach, Charles and I spent the long humid Virginia summers hoeing, weeding, mulching, picking, and selling vegetables. Some farm chores are part of the past; now we mulch every crop to keep weeds down, so there's hardly any hoeing, but I spent many dusty hours hoeing rocky pumpkin fields back then. Other lost tasks I think of more fondly. On the mulch run we brought home scratchy hay bales from local farms. You had to be strong to toss them up onto the wagon to the stacker, but today we unroll little round bales like carpets down tomato aisles. It's much more civilized but less romantic.

When I was eight years old, I began to sell our vegetables at roadside stands in the towns near our farm. After my parents dropped me off, I would set up the table, umbrella, and signs, and wait for people to buy our tomatoes, zucchini, and sweet corn. Stand duty was often lonely, and sometimes scary for a young girl, especially when it got dark. More to the point, we couldn't make a living this way—not with sales of $200 here or $157 there. That winter, my parents took part-time jobs—Dad as a handyman, and Mom waiting tables at the Pizza Hut in Leesburg—to make ends meet.

Only one year later, in 1980, the first farmers' market in our area opened in the courthouse parking lot in Arlington, Virginia, and everything changed. We picked and bunched beets and Swiss chard and drove into town. Scores of grateful customers flocked to our vegetables, as if they had waited all their lives for roadside stands to come to the suburbs of Washington, D.C. That summer we took our vegetables to three weekly farmers' markets, and soon we abandoned roadside stands altogether. With farmers' markets, we began to make a modest profit and farming became a lot more fun. Today, my parents are in their midsixties, and they still make a living exclusively from selling at farmers' markets. They sell twenty-eight varieties of tomatoes, a dozen different cucumbers, garlic, lettuce, and many other vegetables at more than a dozen markets a week in peak season.

We never liked the term *back to the landers* for people who gave up city jobs for farm life. How can you go back to a place you've never been? Yet that's what people called us. I always thought of us as farmers, because farm life was all I ever knew. I have no memories of being a professor's daughter with a stay-at-home, intellectual mother, only of my parents coming in wet from the morning corn pick in the very early days farming with the Newcombs. Even now, after living in Washington, Brussels, London, and now New York City, I still think of myself as a farm girl, happiest when I'm around tomatoes and bugs and creeks.

I Am Forced to Eat Homemade Food

MY MOTHER WAS A natural, if amateur, scientist with an interest in biology, nutrition, and babies. She read about the pioneering experiments of Clara Davis in the 1920s and '30s. Davis set out healthy, whole foods for infants and let them eat anything they wanted for months at a time. The smorgasbord included beef, bone marrow, sweetbreads, fish, pineapple, bananas, spinach, peas, milk and yogurt, cornmeal, oatmeal, rye crackers, and sea salt. At any given meal, the choices babies made could be extreme: one baby ate mostly bone marrow; others loved bananas or milk. One occasionally grabbed handfuls of salt. Over time, however, the babies chose a balanced diet, rich in all the essential nutrients, surpassing the nutritional requirements of the day, and they were in excellent health. The nine-month-old boy with rickets drank cod-liver oil (rich in vitamin D) until his rickets was cured; then he ignored it.

The Clara Davis experiments were limited, and to my knowledge, never repeated. Proven or not, the idea made a deep impression on my mother. She believed that anyone, even an uninformed baby or child—perhaps *especially* a baby or child—could feed himself properly on instinct alone if you gave him only healthy foods, and that was how we ate—at home anyway. There was some leeway for junk food on car trips (Oreos were a treat), and on the rare occasions when we ate out, we could order anything we wanted. At home, however, there was only real food, and my parents never told us what to eat or how much or when.

My mother's other nutritional hero was Adelle Davis, the best-selling writer who recommended whole foods and lots of protein. Before dinner, Mom put out carrot, apple, or turnip sticks so we would eat raw fruits and vegetables when we were hungry for a snack. Main dishes were basic American fare: fried chicken, tuna salad, spaghetti, quiche, meatloaf, potato pancakes with homemade applesauce. There were many frugal dishes, such as chicken hearts with onions, and we ate a lot of rice and beans. At dinner we always had several vegetables and a large green salad.

Most of our food was local and seasonal, which is no doubt why I fondly remember the exceptions, such as the boxes of oranges and grapefruit we bought each winter. We drank fresh raw milk from our Jersey, ate bright-orange eggs from our free-ranging chickens, and a couple of times we slaughtered spent laying hens for soup. Our honey came from a local beekeeper. Occasionally, there was venison or blue fish when we let local people hunt or fish on the property. In those days, few farmers nearby were raising meat and poultry for local markets, so we had to buy those foods at the store, but today our beef, bison, lamb, and chicken come from farmers we know.

Above all, we grew truckloads of vegetables. The simple act of picking vegetables for dinner—a pleasure known to all kitchen gardeners, one that feels maternal and generous to me—is positively extravagant on a real farm, where there are acres of fresh things to choose from. In June I might set out from the kitchen with a basket and a rough plan of attack—to find lettuce, zucchini, and young fennel—and come back with a wheelbarrowfull, seduced along the way by the old spinach patch (abandoned in the hot weather) or by a head of green garlic, still too young to sell but irresistible. If I'm feeling lazy, there's no need to go to the fields at all. In the cool, dark basement, beans, eggplant, and peppers sit in baskets, ready for market.

Our berries, lettuce, herbs, and vegetables made a feast of every meal from April to November. In the old, strict days when every penny counted, the first picking, however tiny—a dozen spears of asparagus or two pints of raspberries—went to market, not to the kitchen. But once each crop was in full swing, we ate as much as we wanted. We grew only the best-tasting varieties, such as Earliglow strawberries and Ambrosia melons. What we didn't grow, we bought or bartered for at farmers' markets. In the winter, we ate our own canned tomatoes and frozen red bell peppers. We all ate huge amounts of vegetables—four ears each of buttered corn, giant plates of sliced tomatoes, enormous green salads—and still do. I've never met anyone who eats more vegetables than my family. To me, a half-cup serving of cooked broccoli is silly, a doll's portion.

Everything we ate was homemade. We made whole wheat bread and buckwheat pancakes from fresh flour ground in an electric mill, and apple, beet, and carrot juice in the juicer. Making granola was a weekly chore for us kids. On winter car trips we packed our own food, typically large pots of beans and rice, bread, apples, and peanut butter. The everyday dessert was apple salad with yogurt or mayonnaise, walnuts, coconut, and honey. When we had proper desserts such as vanilla pudding, cherry pie, and strawberry shortcake—which was not often—they were always made from scratch. Portions were big, leftovers prized, and nothing was wasted. Eggshells and vegetable scraps went in a bucket for the chickens.

It all sounds perfect now, but jars filled with blackstrap molasses and homemade granola did not impress me. I wanted American food, the kind normal kids ate. By far the biggest taboo in our house was junk food, and for that very reason it was deeply compelling. When I had stand duty in the town of Purcellville, I made a beeline for the High's convenience store to buy ice cream sandwiches—and told no one. On my eleventh birthday, my parents said I could have anything I wanted for dinner, and I greedily ordered a store-bought cake. I can still taste the faintly metallic neon frosting. Yet I ate it gamely, unwilling to admit that my hideous cake was inferior to the dessert my mother always made on our birthdays: chocolate éclairs with real milk, butter, and eggs, and good chocolate. The first time I laid eyes on an all-you-can-eat salad bar, at the Leesburg Pizza Hut where my mother waited tables that first winter, I ate a bowl of tasty-looking bacon bits with a spoon. They made me very sick—and embarrassed, too. No one told me you don't eat bacon bits—the lowest form of pork, if they aren't imitation bacon made of soy protein—straight.

These wince-inducing memories suggest that the Clara Davis

experiments—sometimes referred to as proving "nutritional wisdom"—work only when all of the choices are good ones. Sure, the baby cured his rickets with cod-liver oil, like a little instinctive scientist, or a wild animal self-medicating by eating certain plants. But Davis gave the babies only good foods to eat. What if the babies could have eaten ice cream sandwiches, neon pink cake frosting, and bacon bits? To my knowledge, no one has tried such an experiment—unless you count our daily exposure to all manner of cheap junk food—but the evidence is not encouraging.

In the short term, at least, availability seems to determine what we eat, rather than instinct for health. Squirrels, given the choice between acorns and chocolate cookies, take the cookies. The natural diet of sheep is grass, but when offered dense carbohydrates—the ovine equivalent of store-bought cake—they will binge until they are listless. Even a modern hunter-gatherer will drink honey until his teeth rot, if he can get enough.

"As stupid as these choices seem, one can't really blame them on a lack of nutritional wisdom," writes Susan Allport in *The Primal Feast*. "During the course of evolution, squirrels, sheep, and humans have rarely encountered large quantities of concentrated, high-energy foods. Why should the food selection mechanisms of animals include protections against overeating these things? Our human tastes for foods evolved and enabled us to survive in the forests and the African savannas where animals were lean and fibrous, food shortages were a fact of life, and sugar came only in the form of ripe fruits and honey, foods that were available only on an intermittent, seasonal basis." It seems that animals and humans both lack brakes for runaway junk-food craving.

Once you grow up, of course, you have to take responsibility for what you eat, and my parents believed in Emersonian self-reliance. When I was ten or so, they decided that Charles and I should learn to cook, and we drew up a dinner and dishes schedule.

We all cooked the same way, building simple meals around our abundant, gorgeous vegetables. The ingredients weren't fancy, and the recipes weren't sophisticated. I loved my night to cook, especially the grown-up feeling of providing for my family, and here and there I made a stab at something original. Once I prepared Chinese noodle soup by boiling vegetables and pasta in water with lots of soy sauce. My mother wasn't impressed—it probably tasted terrible—but I was proud of my creation and the memory of her reaction hits a tender spot. Another time I baked chicken with rosemary. "It's good," said Charles, "except for the pine needles." My cheeks flushed with shame for introducing a fancy—and risible—ingredient to plain old chicken. Simplicity was a virtue, and culinary experiments weren't much encouraged.

What *was* prized was the idea of the farm as physical paradise. We were encouraged to sigh with delight over the sound of the spring peepers, the flash of the fireflies, the scent of honeysuckle, and—most of all—the flavor of our own melons and tomatoes. I was already a nature lover and took huge pleasure in our beautiful farm and unsurpassed vegetables. But I never understood how appreciation of nature conflicted with making dinner a bit different—tastier, fancier, sexier. Wasn't nice food also a gift of nature?

Now it's obvious that I lived in a kind of paradise about food. My mother's philosophy—provide good homemade food on a budget and then leave your kids alone to eat what they like—was working. Charles and I were healthy, physically active, never picky eaters like other kids we knew—yet looked down on. As for me, it all seemed simple. We grew the best vegetables in the world. At home there was only good stuff, which I ate happily. From time to time, there were treats—like Danish butter cookies—or compelling, but quite possibly regrettable, stuff in restaurants. Mostly, I was ignorant about the big world of food and therefore unashamed. When the school principal sent me home with a free turkey for Christmas, it seemed like nothing more than a stroke of good luck. If my parents didn't care that we didn't have a lot of money and ate simple food, why should I? Above all, I wasn't neurotic about food or my body or my appetites. An untroubled child with lots of energy, I ate what I wanted, when I was hungry for it. Naturally, it didn't last.

My Virtuous Diet Makes Me Plump and Grumpy

A TYPICAL TEENAGE GIRL, I was anxious about all sorts of things, and placed my anxiety squarely on—what else?—food. The experts said that many of the foods I grew up on—like Yorkshire pudding topped with a pool of hot butter—were unhealthy. The smart advice was to be a little bit more vegetarian: eat less meat, less dairy, less saturated fat.

The medical wisdom began to dovetail with our somewhat alternative subculture. Our farming friends and the college students who worked on our farm each summer were health-conscious and green. In those circles, being a vegetarian—better yet, a vegan—was environmentally, nutritionally, and ethically correct. In the worker kitchen down by the little pond, the famous vegetarian *Moosewood Cookbook* was the bible, and communion was rice and beans. Times have changed. Now the workers buy raw milk, eat local venison, and dream of keeping chickens, goats, and cows on their own farms.

The ecological and political arguments for a vegetarian diet came to the fore in 1971, the year I was born. In her seminal book, *Diet for a Small Planet*, Frances Moore Lappé argued that modern beef farming was ecologically unsound (it wrecks natural habitats), politically unjust (you could feed more people on the grain cattle ate than on the steaks), and nutritionally unnecessary (we don't need all that protein). The idea that a vegetarian diet was healthier clinched it for me, and I became a vegan in high school. It was perhaps my only act of rebellion against my stubbornly tolerant parents. My state of mind is still vivid. With all the bad press animal foods were getting, the quickest route to salvation seemed clear: eat only plants.

The summer of 1989 was the last season I lived and worked on the farm. In late August, still the height of the season, my parents drove me to Oberlin College, with the stereo shelf my mother built and my other things in the back of a pickup. Later I transferred to Georgetown University and set up house with my boyfriend in Washington, D.C. In my own kitchen, I was free to invent my own philosophy about food. But I'd lost my instincts and didn't trust my appetite. Eating became an intellectual question. How many people could you feed on the grain it took to raise one steak? If saturated fats are dangerous, why eat any? The vegan experiment ended fairly quickly—I *liked* yogurt—but for many years I was a vegetarian.

Fear of fat and cholesterol dominated our little kitchen in the row house on Twenty-seventh Street in northwest Washington. Even a hint of slippery, creamy food on the tongue sent me into panicky disapproval. Peering at labels, I stocked the pantry with low-fat foods. In those days, I believed the conventional nutritional wisdom: that unsaturated fats were good for cholesterol and saturated fats were not. Monounsaturated olive oil—the star of the vaunted Mediterranean diet—was the only fat I trusted . . . but not much of it. The taboo on cholesterol and saturated fats meant no beef, eggs, cream, chocolate, or coconut. Our only dairy was nonfat yogurt, and there was plenty of rice milk and soy ice cream.

MY VIRTUOUS DIETS

At the height of my various nutritionally correct diets (vegan, vegetarian, low fat, low saturated fat, and low cholesterol), this was the picture:

Real Foods Off the Menu

Beef, lamb, game, poultry, fish, and shellfish
Milk, cream, butter, cheese, and eggs
Chocolate and coconut

Real (But Rich) Foods Strictly Limited

Olive oil
Avocados
Nuts

Real Foods I Ate Plenty Of

Fruits and vegetables
Brown rice and beans
Whole wheat bread

New Foods I Tried to Love

Various imitation foods made with soy and rice

Fat-Free, Sweet Things I Ate Quite a Lot Of

Juice
Nonfat frozen yogurt

Today it's hard to picture *what* we ate. I loved to cook, but most foods were off the menu—no beef, pork, lamb, chicken, fish, milk, or eggs. We ate lots of fresh local vegetables, large green salads, burritos, and bean soups. I ate mountains of rice, beans, and pasta. For dessert there was fruit salad, but without the mayonnaise of my youth. A well-used recipe for nonfat oatmeal bars with pineapple springs to mind, and on special occasions I made fruit pies with butter crust. Now and then I grated low-fat cheese over salad or treated us to grilled shrimp from the waterfront fishmonger.

Now it's clear why my boyfriend gave me a cookbook on my nineteenth birthday: the poor fellow was desperate for variety. It was *Martha Stewart's Quick Cook Menus*, and I read it from cover to cover in one sitting, fascinated with the fancy foods she touted, like balsamic vinegar, crème fraîche, and homemade mayonnaise. Now Martha Stewart is famous for all the domestic arts, from antique paints to pine cone crafts, but in those days she was a champion of simple, seasonal meals—and her recipes always worked. *Quick Cook* was my first cookbook, it bears the marks of many good meals, and I still use it.

As for my health, I felt terrible. My digestion was poor, and I was moody, tearful, and tender in all the wrong places before I got my period. In cold and flu season, I got both. I was depressed, too. Partly to stave off the gloom, I ran three to six miles a day, six days a week. On this virtuous regime I also gained weight steadily—and before I knew it, I was plump. How plump? Well, women and weight is a treacherous topic; no one agrees on the definitions and people get touchy, so I'll try to be objective. I'm almost five feet five inches tall and weigh 119 to 125 pounds, much of it muscle. In my vegetarian days, I was 147 pounds and soft all over. That's a body mass index (BMI) of almost 25, squarely in the "overweight" category.[1]

Back home on the farm in Wheatland, meanwhile, my omnivorous parents were the healthiest people I knew, lean and cheerful as they tucked into fried eggs and pork chops. Something was wrong with me, but I certainly didn't suspect my perfect diet. In

1995, in this none-too-healthy, somewhat muddled state, I moved to Brussels to work for NATO's parliamentary arm. I was twenty-three going on twenty-four, it was my first time going to Europe, and I was full of anxiety. My friend Indya had to reassure me, "There are vegetarians in Europe."

In London I Am Rescued by Farmers' Markets

ON JULY 4, 1996, after a year in Brussels, I moved to England as a journalist for *Time* magazine and found a place on St. Paul Street in Islington, a groovy north London neighborhood. A typical London row house, it had a little, overgrown garden, which I cleared out, hauling away many buckets of shattered concrete from an old patio. A farmer from Cambridgeshire delivered a load of well-rotted compost, which I had fun digging under. I laid a stone path to a spot where the morning sun fell, and put a bench there. One other place got sun, and there I built a raised bed, barely four feet square, for zucchini, herbs, and lettuce. It was a tiny patch, nothing like sixty acres in Virginia, but it was mine.

Apart from the clouds, I loved everything about England and made lots of friends, but soon I was homesick—not for Virginia but for local produce. My sunny patch was too small for all the vegetables I wanted to grow. I tried several whole foods shops and what they call "box schemes" (a weekly delivery), but they all disappointed. The produce was organic, but it was often wilted, bland—and imported. I took the Tube to London's famous street markets, which, not long ago, featured local produce from Kent ("the Garden of England"), but they mostly sold Dutch peppers and Israeli tomatoes and T-shirts.

Imported fruits and vegetables couldn't compare to the ones we grew at home. I longed for ripe strawberries in season, fresh asparagus with its scales unfolding, and traditional apples instead of the standard commercial fare: underripe Granny Smiths from Australia or insipid Red Delicious from Washington State. Desperate for good produce, I rented a site near my house, set about finding farmers, and opened London's first farmers' market on June 6, 1999. The minister of agriculture rang the opening bell, Prince Charles (a keen organic farmer) sent a letter of congratulations, and all the major papers and the BBC turned up. The farmers, many of whom had never sold at retail, were doing a roaring trade. Soon they wanted more markets, and people in other neighborhoods were calling. By September, I'd opened two more, in Notting Hill and Swiss Cottage. In January 2000, I quit my job—by this time I was a speechwriter for the U.S. ambassador to Britain—to start more farmers' markets.

After many years as a fairly dedicated vegetarian, I had begun to eat fish, partly because I had a great fishmonger, but probably more because the experts said fish was good for you. In 1999, a terrific book on brain chemistry, *Potatoes Not Prozac*, persuaded me to eat eggs again and to cut back on juice, honey, and white flour. Very quickly, I felt better and began to need new, smaller clothes. But I was still fat- and cholesterol-wary, quite afraid that meat, butter, and eggs would give me a heart attack.

My own farmers' markets rescued me. Here was real food on my doorstep, just like at home—only better, because there were also new foods I'd never eaten: dried beef, pork pie, crème fraîche. Overnight I stopped using the supermarket, except for things like olive oil, chickpeas, and chocolate. For *The Farmers' Market Cookbook*, I wrote recipes for beef, lamb, pork, poultry, even rabbit—and ate them all. Without really trying, I stopped thinking about food and started tasting it. Beef and lamb didn't thrill me (nor do they now), but I loved roast chicken and bacon. I never meant to lose weight, only to eat more real foods (more ice cream, less nonfat yogurt) and tastier ones (more chicken, less tofu). The pounds did their proverbial melting as I swapped rice and beans for roast chicken, bacon, and cheese.

My other complaints disappeared too, along with the colds and flu. As a vegetarian, I would have scoffed at the idea that my diet was anything but ideal. Now it's clear my body was depleted of protein, saturated fat, fish oil, and vitamins A, B, and D. Among other virtues, protein and fish help keep you trim, B vitamins and fish prevent depression, vitamin A aids digestion, and saturated fats boost immunity. I knew nothing about that, of course, only that the more meat, fish, butter, and eggs I ate, the better I felt. Health and good cheer restored, I became curious about the claims for a vegan and vegetarian diet. What I learned surprised me: we are not natural vegetarians—and no traditional culture is vegan.

Humans are omnivores, meant to eat everything from leaves and fruit to meat and eggs. Our anatomy is a hybrid of the herbivore and carnivore, with flat molars to chew vegetables *and* sharp teeth to tear into meat. Our digestive tract is neither very short (like a dog's) nor very long (like a cow's), but somewhere in between. All over the world, omnivores eat different foods: fish on the coasts, caribou in the woods, beef on the range. But dinner for a cow (grass) or a tiger (meat) is the same everywhere.

For about three million years, we ate mostly animal foods—as a percentage of calories, much more than today. Early humans had a particular taste for bone marrow, brain, fish, and organ meats—and with reason. Marrow contains monounsaturated fats, brain is rich in polyunsaturated fats, fish is the only source of vital omega-3 fats, and liver has loads of iron and vitamins.

This preference for rich food—rather than the leaves and bark other primates ate—had a profound effect, turning us into *Homo sapiens*: the thinking ape. Relative to body weight, we have the biggest brains of all animals. Our brains grew bigger rapidly, easily outpacing more vegetarian primates, says William Leonard, a professor of anthropology at Northwestern University. "Brain expansion almost certainly could not have occurred until hominids adopted a diet sufficiently rich in calories and nutrients."[2] With primates, the general rule is: the bigger the brain, the richer the diet.

We humans are the extreme example of this relationship. Modern hunter-gatherers get 40 to 60 percent of calories from animal fat and protein, compared with a mere 5 to 7 percent for chimps. Our brain is not only big but also ravenous, using sixteen times more energy than muscle by weight. What does the brain need to run smoothly? Fats, especially fish oil. The brain is an astonishing 60 percent fat, of which half is docosahexaeonic acid (DHA).[3] DHA is found only in fish.

The simple truth is this: there are no traditional vegan societies. People everywhere search high and low for animal fat and protein because they are nutritionally indispensable. Frugal cooks use small amounts of meat and fat to supplement the vegetables, grains, and beans that provide most of the calories. Think of collard greens with fatback in the American South, Latino refried beans with lard, and the Asian stir-fry with a little pork and lots of rice. Cooks know that gelatin-rich bone broth extends the poor or scant protein in plants. Even vegetarian societies prize dairy and eggs. Indian cuisine relies on eggs, yogurt, and ghee (clarified butter); Hindus call foods cooked in ghee *pukka* (authentic or superior) and foods in vegetable oil *kachcha* (inferior).

The vegan diet is unnatural and rare because it's risky, especially for babies, children, and pregnant and nursing women. "When women avoid all animal foods, their babies are born small, they grow very slowly and they are developmentally retarded," said Lindsay Allen, director of the U.S. Human Nutrition Research Center. "There's no question that it's unethical for parents to bring up their children as strict vegans."[4] Vegans risk deficiency of three critical nutrients: protein, vitamins, and fish oil.

The body uses protein for structure (muscle, bone, blood) and operations (enzymes made of protein run the whole body). A cow can live on grass, but omnivores need complete protein and they must get it daily because it cannot be stored. Most plants contain some protein—some, like beans, a fair amount—but all plant protein is incomplete. Protein is made of twenty amino acids, nine of which are called *essential* because the body cannot make them. All plants lack one or more of the twenty amino acids, or contain too little of one. Soybeans, for example, have all the amino acids but not enough methionine; corn needs more lysine and tryptophan. Protein needs are unforgiving: when the diet lacks amino acids, the body ransacks its own tissue to find them.

Incomplete plant proteins can be combined to make complete protein. Famous pairs are wheat and milk and rice and beans. Yet this is still second-best nutritionally, for even when combined, plant protein is always inferior to animal protein, in quantity (there's more protein per calorie in fish than in rice and beans) and in quality. Unlike plants, meat, fish, milk, and eggs contain amino acids in the *ideal* amounts for human health.

VEGETARIAN MYTHS

Myth: Our primate cousins are vegetarians.
Truth: All primates eat some animal fat and protein. We eat more to feed our big brains.
Myth: We are natural herbivores.
Truth: We are omnivores with bodies designed to eat plant and animal foods.
Myth: Historically we ate less meat.
Truth: Historically we were even more carnivorous than today.

Myth:	Other cultures are vegan.
Truth:	There are no traditional vegan societies. Even vegetarian cultures use butter and eggs.
Myth:	We don't need animal protein.
Truth:	Omnivores need complete protein every day. A small amount will do.
Myth:	Plant protein is as good as animal protein.
Truth:	Plant protein, even when combined to provide all the amino acids, is inferior to the protein in meat, fish, dairy, and eggs.
Myth:	Soybeans contain complete protein.
Truth:	Soybeans contain all the amino acids but not enough of one (methionine).

Sources: Loren Cordain, *The Paleo Diet*; Weston A. Price Foundation; Joann Grohman, *Real Food*; and www.beyondveg.com.

Deficiency of essential vitamins is a risk of plant-based diets. Vitamin B_6 is found in small amounts in plants, while chicken, fish, and liver are rich sources; vitamin B_{12} is found only in animal foods.[5] Only animal foods (especially seafood, liver, butter, and eggs) contain true vitamins A and D. Animals can make vitamin A from beta-carotene in grass; cows are particularly efficient. Humans, too, can make vitamin A from beta-carotene, but with much more effort. The conversion requires bile salts, fats, and vitamin E. Babies, children, diabetics, and those with thyroid disorders are poor converters. Humans can make some vitamin D in the skin from cholesterol and sunlight when it hits the skin directly, but many people, surprisingly, don't get enough sunlight, especially people with dark skin.

The gravest risk of a strict vegan or vegetarian diet is deficiency of eicosapentaenoic acid (EPA) and DHA, found only in fish. In theory, the body can make these polyunsaturated fats from plants (flaxseed and walnut oil), but humans, especially babies, aren't very good at it. Loren Cordain, a professor at Colorado State University and an expert in historic diets, says that low DHA in mother or baby causes behavioral, mental, and visual problems in infants. Studies show that vegan breast milk is deficient in DHA.[6] Other risks are low birth weight and premature birth.[7]

I found these facts about vegan and vegetarian diets chilling and felt intensely grateful to my omnivorous mother. If I were pregnant or nursing, I'd eat lots of wild salmon, and if my kids got ideas about being vegan, I'd do my damndest to talk them out of it. An adequate *vegetarian* diet, however, is possible, if it includes complete protein, plenty of flaxseed oil, and vitamins A, B_{12}, B_6, and D. If you must be a vegetarian, do eat butter and eggs for the protein and vitamins and flaxseed oil for omega-3 fats. Better still, eat fish, too.

Back in 1999, I knew nothing of chimp diets or vitamin A or why babies need fish. Farmers' markets, not nutrition textbooks, restored my appetite for real food. As I ate my way through the English landscape, discovering local delights like the unctuous smoked eels of Somerset, I wondered: is there an ideal diet for omnivores? In the 1920s, a Cleveland dentist named Weston Price had the same question.

I Discover Weston Price and His Odd Notions

OF ALL THE SIGHTS at a farmers' market, there's none quite like Susan Planck, hell-bent on selling two truckloads of vegetables in four hours. In her midsixties, my mother is lean and fit, with more energy than her crew of eight workers put together. Though she has often had a scant five hours of sleep, she moves lightly and quickly, hefting a bushel of red peppers here, changing a price there. She calls out: "We've had perfect weather for lettuce . . . This is the last week for strawberries!" My mother has a talent for education. From her signs, handouts, and books-to-borrow, customers can learn about everything from soil minerals to breast-feeding.

She's also a sponge for information, so I wasn't surprised when someone at the Falls Church Farmers' Market brought her an article by Sally Fallon called "Why Broth Is Beautiful." Fallon said that stock from beef, poultry, and fish bones is rich in calcium and other minerals, in a form easily assimilated. Broth is also a protein sparer; it is easy to digest and facilitates digestion of everything else. Because it's tasty and nutritious, broth is a key ingredient for frugal peasants and great chefs alike. Fallon called for a "brotherie" in every town serving veal stock, chicken soup, and beef consommé.

My mother wasted no time buying two copies of Fallon's cookbook, *Nourishing Traditions*, and sent me one in London. Many of the recipes were for classic dishes (pot roast, Dover sole with cream sauce), but it was unusual in other ways. She cooked with sweetbreads, extolled fermented foods, and was keen on raw milk and raw liver. The book had high praise for meat, poultry, game, organ meats, eggs, and dairy from animals raised on grass, as well as wild fish and seafood including roe. Above all, Fallon was madly enthusiastic for saturated fats, especially butter and coconut oil.

Fallon, I learned, had founded the Weston A. Price Foundation, a nonprofit dedicated to the work of Weston Price. Chicken broth sounded pretty good, but I wasn't so sure about butter and lard, so I decided to read the five-hundred-page study Price published in 1939 to see for myself. *Nutrition and Physical Degeneration* is a classic work of anthropology, nutrition, and disease prevention. It's also quite a story, and it made me think again about real food.

Weston Price was born in Ontario in 1870 and raised on a farm. He became a dentist and moved to the United States, where he practiced, did research, and wrote respected dentistry textbooks. Price was dismayed at the health of his American patients. Adults suffered from tooth decay and chronic diseases, including arthritis, osteoporosis, and diabetes. Kids had crooked teeth, deformed faces, asthma, infections, allergies, and behavioral problems. The dentist suspected his patients were malnourished on industrial foods, and set out to examine diets in isolated cultures, where people still ate what he called native foods.

Price went to preindustrial communities from Canada to Papua New Guinea, studying the diets of Gaelic fishermen, Ugandan shepherds, and Swiss dairy farmers. All over, he found people with beautiful teeth, perfectly formed faces, and little or no tooth decay—even though they had no dentists or toothbrushes. They were in fine overall health, with none of the chronic illnesses and diseases he saw at home. When they changed their diets, however, and ate what Price called "the displacing foods of commerce"—the sugar and jam, white flour and white rice, and refined vegetable oils that came on ships with European settlers—their health declined sharply.

People who began to eat industrial foods had crooked, crowded, and cavity-ridden teeth and suffered from chronic and fatal diseases including arthritis and tuberculosis. Children of parents who ate refined foods were born with poorly developed facial structure and other deformities like clubfeet. The facial differences in the photos Price took are striking. The unhealthy faces are narrow and asymmetrical, while the healthy ones are broad and shapely. In nature, symmetry is a signal of good conditions (typically nutrition) during growth and development. The human face is no exception.

Price was curious: what did these people eat to stay healthy?

First, they all ate local foods, which meant the diets in different environments varied widely. The communities were roughly of three types: dairy farmers and shepherds; fishermen; and hunter-gatherers.

In Swiss dairy villages, they ate whole raw milk, cream, and butter; whole-grain rye bread or grains of roasted rye; meat on Sundays; soups made with bone broth; and a few summer vegetables. In India and Tibet, they drank tea with milk and butter from sheep and naks—the female yak. Mountain shepherds in Egypt ate butter, which they also traded for millet with farming tribes from the plains. Herding tribes, such as the Masai in Kenya and the Muhima in Uganda, ate mostly meat, blood, and whole milk.

In fishing communities in the Outer Hebrides, remote islands off Scotland, people ate fish, roe, broth, and whole oats. Baked codfish heads stuffed with oats and chopped fish liver were especially popular. Alaskan Eskimo ate mostly seafood, including roe, seal, and whale. They ate no fruit and few vegetables—just a little kelp, cranberries, flowers, and sorrel preserved in seal oil. South Seas islanders and New Zealand Maori ate fish, shark, octopus, shellfish, and sea worms; wild pig and lard; and coconut, manioc, kelp, and fruit.

Hunter-gatherers all over—from Canada to the Everglades, the Amazon to Australia—had the most diverse diet. They ate game, including liver, glands, blood, and marrow; small animals, birds, and insects; and grains, tubers, and vegetables. Indians in the Canadian Rockies, where temperatures fell to seventy degrees below zero, ate no grains, dairy, fruit, or fish. They feasted on caribou and moose and prized moose adrenal glands. In the Andes, Peruvian tribes ate llamas, alpacas, guinea pigs, potatoes, corn, beans, and quinoa, a native grain. Australian Aborigines scrounged anything they could from the harsh landscape: roots, stems, leaves, berries, grass seeds, and a native pea; birds and eggs; seafood and freshwater fish;

kangaroo and wallaby; and a variety of small animals and insects, including rodents, grubs, and beetles. Price made no effort to disguise his admiration for the resourceful Aborigines.

The dentist hoped to find people who lived on land-based foods alone, but he was disappointed. Even when at war, isolated hill people traded (by night, with special dropoffs) with coastal tribes for dried fish roe. Price knew seafoods were rich in iodine, which prevents goiter, mental retardation, and infertility, and vitamins A and D, which aid the absorption of calcium and phosphorus, but he didn't know about vital omega-3 fats found only in fish.

Price concluded there were four factors common to all the diets: whole foods, especially grains; the lack of refined flour and sugar; abundant meat and fish; and unrefined fats. Meat, fish, and fat were vital. Masai and Inuit were almost pure carnivores, and even the few largely vegetarian groups he found ate insects, grubs, and fish when they could. Diets contained all three types of the natural fats: saturated fats from butter, beef, and coconut oil; monounsaturated fats from bone marrow and lard; and polyunsaturated fats in fish and game.

Though Price didn't draw attention to food preparation methods, they were important in traditional diets. Everyone ate raw foods, especially meat, blood, liver, fish, and milk. Raw foods are rich in vitamins, enzymes, and beneficial bacteria. They all favored fermented foods, including milk, grains, juice, and vegetables. Fermentation, a traditional form of preservation, enhances nutrition and aids digestion.

When Price analyzed the foods in his lab, he found that the traditional diets contained ten times more vitamins A and D than the American diet of his day and vastly more minerals, including calcium, magnesium, phosphorus, iodine, and iron. The Eskimo diet contained forty-nine times more iodine than the foods of the colonists.

BUT WE DON'T EAT GRUBS!

Hunter-gatherer diets (historical and contemporary) include foods we may find unappealing, like whale skin and salmon milt. Many tribes eat fat and protein raw, including blood, liver, and fish. For calcium, they crunch through bones in fish and small birds and savor pungent fermented foods. They eat these foods for vitamins, minerals, and enzymes. Happily, we can get the same nutrients from foods more familiar to the European-American palate. Caesar salad contains raw egg, fermented Parmesan Reggiano, and anchovies, a fermented fish we eat whole, bones and all. Smoked salmon, steak tartare, and mayonnaise are three famous dishes of raw fish, meat, and eggs. Classic eggnog is made with raw egg and raw cream. It's not necessary to eat *exactly* like a hunter-gatherer, only to obtain the nutrients they knew they needed.

Back home, Price set out to cure the unhealthy children in his clinic with good food. Their typical diet contained mostly refined foods: black coffee with sugar, white bread and pancakes, donuts fried in vegetable oil. In one experiment, Price fed malnourished kids one meal daily, six days a week, while they ate as usual at home. The therapeutic meals included liver, fish chowder, or a meat stew made of broth and carrots; a buttered whole wheat roll made with freshly ground flour; tomato juice with cod-liver oil; and two glasses of whole milk. The meat, dairy, and eggs came from animals raised on grass, which Price had found contained more vitamin A than animals raised on grain. It was the American version of the traditional diets: rich in protein, vitamins A, B, and D, omega-3 fats, and minerals. The children's health—and their performance in school—improved sharply. "A properly balanced diet," Price wrote, "is good for the entire body."

THE FERTILITY DIET

In traditional diets, special foods were reserved for couples before conception and for women during pregnancy. Key nutrients include calcium, iodine, zinc, vitamin A, and omega-3 fats. Peruvian tribes in the Andes traveled hundreds of miles to trade with valley tribes for kelp and salmon roe, for iodine, vitamin A, zinc, and omega-3 fats. Alaskan Inuit ate dried fish eggs for fertility, while in North America, Indians ate the iodine-rich thyroid glands of the male moose. In Africa, the largely vegetarian Kikuyu fed girls extra animal fat for six months before marriage. In dairy villages, the fertility diet included raw spring-grass butter for vitamins A and D.

Today doctors tell pregnant women to take folic acid to prevent the birth defect spina bifida, but few couples are advised to eat a preconception diet. The first thing a woman needs to conceive is enough estrogen (in her fat) to ovulate. Men and women who would be parents should eat plenty of foods containing zinc, omega-3 fats, and vitamin A (needed to make estrogen). Eat cod-liver oil and butter, cream, egg yolks, and liver from grass-fed animals. Vitamin E is essential for sperm production; deficiency can cause permanent sterility. Sperm health improves dramatically when vitamins A and E are taken together, probably because vitamin E prevents oxidation of vitamin A. Protein and B vitamins, especially B_{12}, are crucial for egg production, sperm count, and sperm motility. The omega-3 fat DHA is found in high concentrations in sperm.

Nutrition and Physical Degeneration was comprehensive, monumental—and controversial. Dentists and anthropologists welcomed the work—at one time, the book was on the reading list for anthropology classes at Harvard—but most medical professionals ignored it. Price himself noted frequently that his approach to disease was unorthodox. His work did, however, inspire the nutritionist Adelle Davis. Davis had a masters degree in biochemistry from the University of Southern California Medical School, but she wrote about nutrition in a friendly, common-sense style. In the 1950s and '60s, titles like *Let's Eat Right to Keep Fit* and *Let's Get Well* became bestsellers.

Growing up on a farm in Indiana, Davis ate a traditional American breakfast of hot cereal, steak, ham, eggs, sausage, and fried chicken with gravy, all washed down with grass-fed, whole milk—and that was exactly the food she recommended for a diet rich in protein and vitamins A, D, and B. Davis extolled whole grains, unrefined fats, whole milk, and plenty of protein, including beef, liver, fish, and eggs. She called for raw foods, including eggs, liver, and milk. Davis was ahead of her time; she wrote that hydrogenated fats were dangerous and fish oil reduces cholesterol.

Like Price, Davis was controversial. "She so infuriated the medical profession and the orthodox nutrition community that they would stop at nothing to discredit her," recalls my friend Joann Grohman, a dairy farmer and nutrition writer who says Adelle Davis restored her own health and that of her five young children. "The FDA raided health food stores and seized her books under a false labeling law because they were displayed next to vitamin bottles."

Price and Davis were pioneers in the field now known as nutritional epidemiology—the study of nutrition and disease—and modern research confirms their work. The experts now agree, for example, that hydrogenated vegetable oil, not butter, raises LDL.

As we'll see later, heart disease is caused by a diet deficient in B vitamins, not by saturated fats. Researchers even explore the subtle interplay between diet and how genes function. The omega-3 fats EPA and DHA, for example, activate the expression of genes controlling fat metabolism, which may explain how they prevent obesity. Hippocrates gave us the essence of nutritional epidemiology: "Let food be your medicine and medicine be your food."

After I read about traditional diets, it was clear how my vegan, fat-free ways had depleted my body. But one thing was nagging me: whether eating saturated fat and cholesterol every day was really okay. Before I dived headfirst into traditional beef, butter, and eggs, it seemed sensible to find out what modern science had to say about them. I started to do some homework on real food.

Everywhere I Go, People Are Afraid of Real Food

AT THE UNION SQUARE GREENMARKET in New York City, an older woman was buying chicken. "I can't eat any skin," she told the farmer firmly. "This is the best chicken on the market," I chimed in, "because it's raised on pasture. And the skin is good for you too, full of healthy fats." She turned toward me, indignant. "I never eat the skin," she said. "It's bad for you, all that fat!"

At Murray's, the oldest cheese shop in New York City, a young woman was asking for low-fat mozzarella. She prefers whole milk mozzarella, she said, but feels "less guilty" eating the skim milk version.

At home, I serve my friends roast chicken, mashed potatoes with milk and butter, spinach salad with bacon, tart cherry pie with lard crust, and raw whipped cream. "There goes my cholesterol," jokes one of them. "Don't tell my doctor!" Even as they dig into this delicious and satisfying food, they cannot forget that it's going to kill them. "Heart attack on a plate," says another. The tone combines fear, resignation, and guilty pleasure.

All these good people are wrong.

The woman at the farmers' market doesn't know that chicken fat is monounsaturated and polyunsaturated—two fats even the conventional experts say are healthy. Why would she? According to the experts, the less fat the better, and chicken fat is no exception. Schmaltz is a guilty pleasure. Here, the farmer is no help; he doesn't know what's in chicken fat, either. Chickens raised on grass contain more conjugated linoleic acid (CLA), an unusual fat which fights cancer and builds lean muscle. Chicken fat also boosts immunity. The Jewish penicillin wasn't skinless chicken breasts; it was chicken soup, with droplets of golden fat that also make chicken soup silky. But *someone* taught this lady that chicken fat is poison—not her mother, I'll bet—and she's sticking to it.

The young woman at Murray's doesn't know that you need the fat in milk to digest the protein and absorb the calcium. If she struggles with her weight, she may discover—as million of Americans have, after thirty years of dubious advice—that eating foods engineered to be low-fat doesn't work, especially when you eat more calories because the food is unsatisfying. Also, the latest research indicates that milk, yogurt, and cheese actually aid weight loss, perhaps due to the effects of calcium on fat storage.

At my house and at the farm, we eat the way people did for thousands of years. That means all the foods they tell you to avoid: red meat, whole milk, sausage, butter, and raw milk cheese. But the beef and milk are grass-fed, the pork and poultry are pastured, and the fats—from lard to coconut oil—are unrefined. Milk, cream, and butter are grass-fed and raw. I relish the rich, unfashionable cuts you never see in "heart-healthy" diets, such as liver and bone marrow—just as our Stone Age ancestors did. I don't buy low-fat versions of anything. Foods should be eaten with the fats they come with: whole milk, chicken with skin.

All this real food is good for you. How?

- *Grass-fed beef* is rich in beta-carotene and vitamin E (both fight heart disease and cancer) and CLA, the anticancer fat.
- *Grass-fed milk, cream, butter, and cheese* are rich in vitamins A and D, omega-3 fats, and CLA. Butter contains butyric acid, another fat that fights cancer and infections.
- *Pastured pork and lard* are rich in antimicrobial fats and the monounsaturated fat oleic acid—the same fat in olive oil, which reduces LDL.
- *Pastured eggs* are rich in vitamins A and D. They contain omega-3 fats, which prevent obesity, diabetes, heart disease, and depression. Egg yolks contain lecithin, which helps metabolize cholesterol.

Cholesterol. This word alone can stop a story about food in its tracks. The thought of rich, sweet cream has barely taken shape before the evil ingredient cholesterol flutters by, landing smack-dab in the worry corner of the brain to spoil the reverie. I know what you're thinking. *Aren't saturated fats and cholesterol dangerous?* I don't think so.

Let's first agree that Americans are right to be worried about diet and health. Since 1900, once-rare conditions—obesity, diabetes, and heart disease—have become rampant. These three are known as the diseases of civilization, because for most of human history they were all but unheard of. (Three million years ago, if you were obese or diabetic or your heart failed, you would soon be dead.) In the United States today, obesity, diabetes, and heart disease are chronic diseases. They can be deadly, but just as often, they're a condition people live with, thanks to a combination of drugs, surgery, and diminished quality of life—as in "I'm too fat and out of breath to play catch with my dog." People with type 2 diabetes survive on insulin injections. In 1950, most heart attacks were fatal. But today, thanks to major medical advances, more Americans with chronic heart disease are living longer. Certainly, enabling people to live with chronic disease is a sign of progress. Preventing disease is another—the one that interests me.

The reader might object that life in the Stone Age was different. For the hunter-gatherer couple, it was nasty, brutish, and short; he might be gored by a mastodon and she was apt to bleed to death while giving birth. We, on the other hand, live much longer, with ample time to grow old and to develop degenerative diseases. How do we know the meat-loving hunter-gatherers would not have keeled over from hardened arteries, too, had they managed to survive to sixty-five?

Good question. Loren Cordain, an expert in Stone Age diets, looked into this one. In most hunter-gatherer groups, 10 to 20 percent are sixty years or older—and in fine health. "These elderly people have been shown to be generally free of the signs and symptoms of chronic disease (obesity, high blood pressure, high cholesterol levels) that universally afflict the elderly in western societies," he says. "When these people adopt western [industrial] diets . . . they begin to exhibit signs and symptoms of 'diseases of civilization.'" So much for the idea that age equals disease.

Let's next agree that the experts are right: diet does affect blood. The study of blood cholesterol and its various subcategories is getting more sophisticated by the hour, but the conventional wisdom holds that it's better for high-density lipoprotein (HDL) to be high and low-density lipoprotein (LDL) to be low. Casually known as the "good" and "bad" cholesterol hypothesis, this idea emerged when it became clear that the number they call "total cholesterol" was a poor—very poor—predictor of heart disease.

Today, most experts believe that low HDL and high LDL are "risk factors" for heart disease, which means the two conditions are statistically correlated.

But I'm not so sure. There are two important caveats to the rule that high LDL, in particular, is dangerous. The first is a lesson from Statistics 101: correlation does not necessarily imply cause. In other words, high LDL does not necessarily *cause* heart disease. Instead, it could be a symptom (or *marker*, as experts say) of heart trouble. The second caveat is equally serious: many studies show that high LDL and heart disease are *not* linked. In 2005, the *Journal of American Physicians and Surgeons* reported that as many as half of the people who have heart disease have normal or "desirable" LDL.[8] Also in 2005, researchers found that older men and women with high LDL live longer.[9] When the rule—high LDL is dangerous—doesn't apply in the elderly or in half of the heart disease cases, the honest scientist can only conclude one thing: the rule needs a second look. Some cholesterol experts believe the rule needs more than just tweaking. "There is nothing bad about LDL," says Joel Kauffman, Professor of Chemistry Emeritus at the University of the Sciences in Philadelphia. "There never was."[10]

What might account for the inconsistent findings on LDL and heart disease? First, the link some studies show between high LDL and heart disease could be explained by oxidation. Research in humans and animals shows that natural LDL is a normal part of a healthy body, but *oxidized* or damaged LDL is bad news. Perhaps high LDL readings really represent high *oxidized* LDL. Second, does cholesterol really clog arteries? Probably not. According to Kauffman, there is no relationship between total cholesterol (or LDL) and atherosclerosis. As we'll see later, an amino acid called homocysteine, not cholesterol, actually damages arteries.

Later, we'll look at cholesterol in more detail, but for now, let me say this: I believe the "good" and "bad" cholesterol story has failed to explain heart disease fully—and worse, it has failed to prevent it. The narrative of evil LDL and knightlike HDL oversimplifies a complex reality.

What about diet? Other things being equal, does eating foods like butter and eggs, rich in natural cholesterol and natural saturated fat, have an undesirable effect on blood cholesterol and lead to heart disease? From what I can gather, the answer is no. High cholesterol and heart disease are rare in cultures where people eat cholesterol-rich foods, including butter, eggs, and shrimp. The same is true in tropical cultures where they eat saturated coconut oil daily. Studies of traditional diets are only one reason I eat butter, cream, and coconut oil with impunity. Happily, clinical studies confirm this observation about saturated fats.

The story about diet and disease is more complicated than just saturated fats and cholesterol, of course. As we'll see, reductionist thinking is precisely the mistake the experts, who focused everything on cutting fat and cholesterol, made. Traditional diets are also rich in many other nutrients that *prevent* heart disease, including omega-3 fats in fish and B vitamins. But one thing is clear: if beef and butter were to blame for heart disease, heart disease would not be new. We've been eating them for too long.

Look at the traditional diets in the accompanying table. They contain more calories, and many more calories from animal foods, than the modern American diet. Yet Americans are overweight with higher cholesterol levels. Evenki reindeer herders in Russia derive almost half their calories from meat, almost twice as much as the average American. Yet Evenki men are 20 percent leaner than American men, with cholesterol levels 30 percent lower.[11]

MODERN AMERICAN DIET VERSUS TRADITIONAL DIETS

	Inuit in North America	*Evenki shepherds in Russia*	*Modern Americans*
Daily calories	2,350	2,820	2,250
Calories from animal foods (%)	96	41	23
Calories from plant foods (%)	4	59	77
Cholesterol	141	142	204
Body mass index*	24	22	26

* A healthy BMI is 18.5–24.9. Above 25 is overweight, and above 30 is obese.

Source: William R. Leonard, "Food for Thought," *Scientific American*, August 2003, Vol 13, No 2 (updated from the December 2002 issue).

Clearly, the Americans are doing something wrong. Even though we eat fewer calories and more calories from plant foods than the Inuit and Evenki, we're fat and have "high" cholesterol. The fault may well lie in our diets, but judging from these cases—and many similar studies of modern hunter-gatherers such as Australian aboriginals—it's unlikely that saturated animal fat *itself* causes unhealthy cholesterol. These lean, healthy people eat a lot of saturated animal fat. Something else must be to blame for our own poor health.

What might that be? The culprit is industrial foods. Sugar and hydrogenated vegetable oils raise cholesterol and triglycerides. Eating oxidized—or damaged—cholesterol leads to unhealthy oxidized LDL in the body. The main, dietary source of oxidized cholesterol is powdered skim milk and powdered eggs, commonly found in processed foods. Finally, other factors are vitally important. Exercise, for example, keeps you thin and raises HDL. You can bet that Inuit seal hunters and Evenki shepherds get more exercise than most Americans.

The experts are right: our diet is killing us. But traditional beef, butter, and eggs are not to blame for obesity, diabetes, and heart disease. The so-called diseases of civilization are caused by the foods of civilization. More accurately, the diseases of *industrialization* are caused by the foods of *industrialization.*

2

Real Milk, Butter, and Cheese

I Am Nursed on the Perfect Food

ON THE DAY I WAS BORN, at home in our big house on 84 Russell Avenue in Buffalo, New York, my mother and I had everything we wanted. That afternoon she rested comfortably on the couch in our sunny front room, in no particular hurry for anything to happen, with her family checking in occasionally. March 29, 1971 fell on a Monday, but my father didn't go to work and my sister and brother stayed home from school. The doctor was just taking off her coat when I arrived on a schedule known only to my mother and me. Then my mother fed me the perfect food from the perfect container. Later, she fed herself some real food: mail order organic beef liver from Walnut Acres, one of the pioneering organic brands.

I was a lucky baby. My mother gave me real food in my first hours and nursed me on demand until I stopped asking for fresh raw milk three years later. If possible, a woman should nurse exclusively for at least one year, or, ideally, until the baby loses interest. Though it's uncommon today among working women, nursing longer than the usual six or twelve months is natural. In modern hunter-gatherer societies, nursing for three years is typical and four to six years is not unheard of. UNICEF and the World Health Organization advise breast-feeding for "two years and beyond."

Breast-feeding cements a profound bond between mother and baby. When things are going well, by all accounts, it's a very nice sensation. Mothers describe loving, trancelike feelings when nursing, and babies will suckle long after they are full. In *Fresh Milk: The Secret Life of Breasts,* Fiona Giles collected memories of nursing from young children. "It was comforting and relaxing," said an eight-year-old boy. "I looked forward to it." A twelve-year–old girl was more blunt: "The word *addictive* comes to mind." An older sibling who had been weaned acted out her own farewell as she watched the new baby nurse. She would cover her mother's breasts and say, "Bye bye, delicious milk."

Breast milk is our first food, the best food, the ultimate traditional food in all cultures without exception. That's why nature made nursing satisfying: to encourage mothers and babies to do it.

Because it was designed as the baby's only source of food, breast milk is a complete meal. If the mother is well nourished on real food, her breast milk will contain just the right amount of protein, fat, carbohydrates, and all the other nutrients for the growing baby, including essential vitamins, with one notable—and interesting—exception. The milk of all mammals lacks iron. Moreover, milk contains the protein lactoferrin, which ties up any random iron that does find its way into the young. There is logic in the missing iron: iron is necessary for the growth of *E. coli*, the most common source of infant diarrhea in all species. A breast-fed baby rarely needs any additional iron before one year; bottle-fed babies may need iron sooner because infant formula depletes iron. After one year, iron-rich raw liver is often the first solid food for babies in traditional diets.

Breast milk is not only a complete meal but also a rich one: about 50 percent of its calories come from fat. Indeed, fats may be the most important thing about breast milk. At the most basic level, fat is essential for the baby's growth and development, and for assimilating protein and the fat-soluble vitamins A and D, but each particular fat in breast milk also plays an important role.

The long-chain polyunsaturated omega-3 fats EPA and DHA in mother's milk are vital to eye and brain development in the baby. Pregnant and nursing women should eat plenty of fish—the only source of fully formed EPA and DHA—and keep eating it. With each pregnancy, a woman's store of omega-3 fats is depleted. The hungry baby neither knows nor cares whether her mother eats wild salmon, but simply takes the omega-3 fats she needs to build her own brain.

As we saw earlier, vegans and vegetarians risk deficiency of EPA and DHA. The breast milk of vegan mothers contains less DHA than nonvegan breast milk.[1] Nursing mothers who do not eat fish are wise to take a generous supplement of flaxseed oil. The body *can* make EPA and DHA from flaxseed oil, but the conversion is uncertain and imperfect. It bears repeating: fish is vastly superior to plant sources of omega-3 fats.

Most of the fat in breast milk is saturated. The body needs saturated fat to assimilate the polyunsaturated omega-3 fats and calcium. Mother's milk is a rare source of a saturated fat called lauric acid. Antimicrobial and antiviral, lauric acid is so critical to the baby's immunity that it must, by law, be added to infant formula; the usual source is coconut oil.

The ample cholesterol in human milk is essential to the developing brain and nervous system. So vital is cholesterol, breast milk contains a special enzyme to ensure the baby absorbs it fully.[2] Humans make cholesterol in the liver and brain, but infants and children do not make enough cholesterol for health. Thus the American Dietetic Association says the diets of children under two must include cholesterol.[3]

Many other factors in breast milk boost the baby's immunity, an essential shield in its new, germ-filled world. White blood cells, sugars called oligosaccharides, and lactoferrin fight bacteria and viruses. (Lactoferrin from human milk is patented for use in killing *E. coli* in the meatpacking industry.) Mother's milk contains all five of the major antibodies, especially IgA, which is found throughout the human digestive and respiratory systems and protects tissues from pathogens.[4] Babies don't begin to make their own IgA for weeks.

In one of nature's many elegant efficiencies, the antibodies in breast milk are targeted to the pathogens in the mother and baby's immediate environment; they are tailor-made for the baby. Dr. Jack Newman, a breast-feeding consultant to UNICEF, says researchers can't explain "how the mother's immune system knows to make antibodies against only pathogenic and not normal bacteria, but whatever the process may be, it favors the establishment of 'good bacteria' in a baby's gut."

BREAST MILK: A COMPLETE MEAL

- Complete protein and carbohydrate (for growth)
- Saturated lauric acid (to fight infection)
- Polyunsaturated EPA and DHA (for the brain and eyes)
- Cholesterol (for brain and nerves)
- Many immune factors (to fight infections)
- Beneficial bacteria (for digestion)

Breast milk is the most important food a mother will ever feed her baby. A convincing number of studies confirm that babies who drink this perfect food tend to have better immunity and digestion, lower mortality, and higher IQ than formula-fed infants. They typically have lower rates of hospital admissions, pneumonia, stomach flu, ear and urinary tract infections, and diarrhea than bottle-fed babies. In later life, breast-fed babies often have lower blood pressure and cholesterol, and extra protection against juvenile rheumatoid arthritis, asthma, allergies, respiratory infections, eczema, immune system cancers such as lymphoma, Crohn's disease, diabetes, stroke, and heart disease. Breast-fed babies are less likely to be obese when they grow up, possibly because breast milk is rich in the protein adiponectin. Adiponectin lowers blood sugar and affects how the body burns fat. Low levels of adiponectin are linked to obesity, type 2 diabetes, and heart disease.

Some women find that breast-feeding is not as easy as it looks in those lovely paintings of Madonna and Child. For many understandable reasons, mother and baby may find nursing difficult, painful, or in extreme cases impossible. If nursing isn't right for you and your baby, choose a formula with care. Even with the best intentions, it hasn't been easy for scientists to duplicate the properties of breast milk, which contains more than three hundred known ingredients and probably still more yet to be identified. Most formula contains a mere forty ingredients, and often the main ingredient is sugar. In the United States, most infant formula contains no long-chain polyunsaturated omega-3 fats, an unconscionable omission given their vital role in the eyes and brain. The World Health Organization and the European Union both recommend omega-3 fats for babies; infant formula with DHA is widely available in Europe and Asia.

Soy-based formula and low-fat diets are particularly unwise for babies and children. As we'll see later, soy is far too rich in estrogens. Low-fat diets cause stunted growth, learning disabilities, interrupted sexual development, and the syndrome seen in the babies of malnourished vegan and vegetarian mothers, "failure to thrive," which is marked by slow growth and lethargy.[5]

The best substitute for breast milk is made from grass-fed, raw whole milk, supplemented with live yogurt cultures and gelatin (for digestion), coconut oil (for immunity), and cod-liver oil (for the eye and brain).[6] There are also human milk banks for special cases, such as premature babies and those who are allergic to formulas. Throughout history, women, including wet nurses, have provided milk for infants whose own mothers were unwilling or unable to do so. At the Mother's Milk Bank in Austin, Texas, potential donors are carefully screened with blood tests, and donated milk is pasteurized and tested before being fed to babies.

Traditional societies provide advice and assistance to nursing mothers, usually from older relatives or experienced local women. The contemporary equivalent of this support network is La Leche League, an excellent and friendly source of practical and scientific knowledge about breast-feeding. If you are nursing and run into difficulty, or if you feel lonely or discouraged, try calling these modern-day wise women. They know all about cracked and tender nipples—and your baby will thank you one day.

I Remember Milking Mabel the Cow

WHEN I WAS TWO YEARS OLD, we moved to the Newcombs' farm in Fairfax County, Virginia, and thus began our relationship with a long line of family cows. There was a red and white Hereford named Katy, a gentle black Angus called Steady Teddy, and then the milk cows: a Guernsey named Emma, who slipped out one evening and was never heard from again, and a Jersey called Tai Tai—an honorific akin to "Mrs." in Mandarin. Later, when we moved to our own farm in Loudoun County, we bought Mabel, a chocolate-colored Jersey. I'm afraid her character didn't conform to the stereotype of the docile cow. My brother, Charles, remembers that "Mabel was often irritated with us."

By then I was nine or ten, and milking was one of my regular chores. On my night to milk, I'd bring Mabel into the barn from the pasture, put her in the stanchion, and give her a little grain while I washed her udder. Then I'd sit on a wooden stool my brother had helped me build and begin to milk, making a ring with my thumb and forefinger and squeezing the teat from the top down, one finger at a time, first one hand, then the other.

There is a pleasant, lulling rhythm to milking. Even now the sounds are vivid: Mabel's noisy chewing and breathing, the soft rustling as the chickens settled in for the night. At first, when the bucket is empty, the milk goes "ping" as it hits the tin. As the pail fills up, each squirt meets the foamy liquid and the pitch drops. In the summer, her tail—called a *switch* in dairy lore—might miss the flies on her flank and sting my face. With Mabel, there was also a good chance she'd lose her poise and kick the bucket over or step right in it. You had to whisk the bucket away.

Before long her bag was loose and empty, and there were a couple of gallons of milk. If she'd been scratched by brambles, I rubbed her udder with a miraculous salve called Bag Balm, made in Lyndonville, Vermont, since 1899. (I still use it on my own cuts and scratches.) I carried the milk across the footbridge to the house and strained it through a striped pink cloth into glass gallon jars. We wrote the date, plus AM or PM, on masking tape and stuck it to the jar. That was it.

Going to school smelling of cow was mortifying, and when I had to milk in the morning I always took my shower afterward. I knew we weren't supposed to *sell* raw milk—after we put an ad in the paper, two friendly women from the state came around to tell us to keep it quiet—but was ignorant about why it was better than supermarket milk. The jars of milk in the fridge were like the wheat berries on the shelves: embarrassing.

Eventually the burden of daily milking grew tedious, and we sold Mabel to a local man, luring her into his truck with sweet corn, and we never kept a cow again. It seems sad now. Having visited dairy farms small and large, tasted industrial and real milk side by side, and learned a bit about how butter and cheese are made, I begin to grasp that having more fresh milk and cream than we could drink was a luxury.

Historically, milk was more than a luxury; it was critically important in the diet. For peasants, the cow kept the grocery bill down and the doctor away. With her ability to convert inedible grass into milk and cream, the cow was at the center of the domestic economy. Rich in protein, fat, calcium, and B vitamins, milk was known as "white meat," capable of transforming an inadequate diet of bread and potatoes into a passable one, especially for children. In *cucina povera* (peasant cooking), vegetables are often soaked in milk before roasting.

A cow needs nothing more than a patch of grass, but most European peasants were too poor to own land, and for centuries they grazed animals on common land. In Britain and elsewhere, the gradual loss of access to the commons in the late eighteenth century was catastrophic for peasants, who were no longer able to keep cattle for milk and meat. The British historian J. M. Neeson describes "the stubborn memory of roast beef and milk" and their "swift disappearance" from the diet of the poor after the loss of grazing rights.[7] In 1786, the cleric H. J. Birch wrote that butter was too dear for his Danish parishioners. They made do with bread crusts, beer, and cabbage boiled without meat. When "cottagers receive not the smallest patch of land or grazing for cows or sheep, and are not even entitled to keep as much as a couple of geese on the common . . . then poverty and need reach dire extremes; then cottagers begin to beg—people who have never begged before, and never thought of begging."[8]

In the New World, too, milk was a staple, from the earliest colonial days right through the middle of the twentieth century, when farmers like my great-aunt Esther still kept a cow in Milford,

Illinois. Esther and Uncle Charlie mostly raised crops, but they most likely made a little extra money selling milk and cream. Initially, colonial Americans preferred goats, probably because they were rugged and good at clearing land, and by 1639 there were four thousand goats in the Massachusetts Bay Colony. But the cow—a superior milker—gradually replaced goats. Oxen also pulled the plow and provided beef and leather.

Though grazing was allowed on public sites like Boston Common, the European model of using common land for grazing wasn't widespread. The self-sufficient homestead was the original American dream and became the typical farming pattern. In 1626, each family in the Plymouth Colony was allotted one cow and two goats for every six shares of land they held. "This ideal characterized small farming in America for another two centuries," write Annie Proulx and Lew Nichols in *The Complete Dairy Foods Cookbook*.

JERSEY, QUEEN OF COWS

I'm charmed by the colorful names of breeds, suggesting their hometown (Kerry) or looks (Dutch Belted) or qualities (Milking Devon). Others known for milk, meat, or both include the Hereford, Simmental, Limousin, Angus, Brown Swiss, Ayrshire, Milking Shorthorn, Norwegian Red, and Holstein-Friesian. The star of the industrial dairy is the Holstein, a Dutch cow known for copious production of low-fat, watery milk. For small dairies, the undisputed champion is the Jersey, a small cow native to the Channel Islands. Docile, an efficient grazer even on poor pasture, intelligent, and productive, she is also the ideal family cow. But the Jersey's crowning glory is her milk: it contains the highest level of protein, minerals, vitamins, and

> butterfat of any breed. Jersey milk is 5 to 6 percent butterfat, nearly twice as rich as Holstein milk, with 3 to 3.5 percent fat—the norm for whole milk. Jersey milk (and that of her cousin, the Guernsey) is too rich for some to drink straight. No matter; there will be plenty of fat for cream, butter, and cheese.

Today the family cow is rare, but her role is the same. "The cow is the most productive, efficient creature on earth," writes Joann Grohman in *Keeping a Family Cow*. "She will give you fresh milk, cream, butter, and cheese, building health, or even making you money. Each year she will give you a calf to sell or raise for beef." The cow also provides manure for the garden, sour milk for the chickens, and skim milk or whey for the pig—milk-fed pork being a delicacy. "I serve exceptionally fine food"—I can confirm this, having eaten at Joann's house—"and I am not stingy with the butter and cream," says Grohman. "The cow is a generous animal."

Keeping a Family Cow inspired Laura Grout, a mother of five, to change her life. "I was living in a trailer park with a postage stamp for land and researching nutrition. After learning that unpasteurized milk is better for your health, I went looking for a legal way to obtain raw milk. This book alone convinced me to leave the city and have a cow." Laura began to raise her own beef, milk, poultry, and eggs in Sand Hollow, Idaho. "Good nutrition is something every mother should strive to give her children," she says, "no matter how rich or poor."[9]

That was my mother's philosophy in a nutshell. She used to say, "No matter how little money we spend on food, we will always have maple syrup, olive oil, and butter." Now that I live in the city and pay good money for real milk and cream, the significance of a cow is tangible: Mabel made us richer. I loved a bowl of milk and mashed-up peaches; we put milk on hot oatmeal, and dessert was often vanilla pudding or custard. After school, Charles and I made smoothies with raw milk, eggs, coffee, and honey. With Mabel, milk was free and life was good.

A Short History of Milk

OVER THOUSANDS OF YEARS, humans have herded, corralled, and milked a variety of mammals. In the Near East, our ancestors domesticated sheep and goats about eleven thousand years ago; archaeologists surmise that milk, not meat, was the initial reason for keeping animals. The first shepherds tended sheep and goats, small and easy to handle. They are also rugged: they thrive on poor farmland and don't mind harsh climates. Sheep tolerate cold, wind, and snow, while goats scamper up the steepest mountain and live off brambles or any weed that happens to grow in hedgerows. On the rocky slopes of Greece and the hills of hot, dry Provence, sheep milk cheese (salty, crumbly feta) and goat milk cheese (creamy chèvre) have been made since ancient times.

About eighty-five hundred years ago, somewhere in Mesopotamia (modern Iraq), we began to milk the larger and more productive cow. Cows are more delicate than sheep and goats—in bad weather they prefer the barn, and for grazing they favor lush rolling pasture—yet of all the mammals humans have tried, including asses, buffalo, camels, llamas, mares, reindeer, and yaks, the cow is the champion milker.

That's the conventional chronology of milking, at any rate, but several clues suggest we were drinking milk for much longer than ten thousand years. One clue lies in the popular understanding, or misunderstanding, of early agricultural history. Most people believe that "farming" (meaning both plant and animal husbandry) began about ten thousand years ago in the Fertile Crescent. It is more likely, however, that we herded animals long before we grew corn, wheat, and beans. There is no *agricultural* reason to link milking with growing grains. The natural diet of ruminants is grass. Early shepherds didn't need to grow grain: they needed only meadows and some skill in handling animals.

Fences imply that we were shepherds before we were farmers. "Thirty thousand years ago, people in the High Sinai were confining and breeding antelope with the aid of fences, a human invention arguably as important as the spear," writes Grohman in *Keeping a Family Cow*. Fences were the best means of keeping the best milkers close at hand and choosing the most docile and productive cows to mate. The friendly, efficient dairy cow has been the focus of so much intensive breeding over thousands of years that today she has no wild cousins left, and lives only at our whim.

All meat and dairy cattle are descendants of the original wild ox, a six-thousand-pound giant called an aurochs, described by Julius Caesar as only slightly smaller than an elephant. "The aurochs became extinct in the seventeenth century, the last one dying alone in a private park in Poland," writes Gina Mallet in *Last Chance to Eat*. "But it can be seen depicted in cave paintings: a large, bony animal with sharp horns impaling stick humans." How the fierce aurochs—a symbol of strength in Viking runes—was eventually domesticated is a mystery. In *A Cow's Life*, M. R. Montgomery suggests that Neolithic man tamed an aurochs midget first.

In time we were master of bull and cow alike. Fish and game made up most of the typical Paleolithic diet, but this new food, milk, had its advantages and before long it was popular. As a source of daily protein, milking wild ruminants was more reliable than hunting, which was hit-or-miss. Hunting also presented a practical problem. Because it was impossible to keep meat fresh without refrigeration, fresh kill had to be eaten quickly. The immediate family of the successful hunter couldn't eat a wooly mammoth in one sitting, so the bounty was shared with the tribe or village. Thus sharing meat with other men—or trading meat (dinner) for sex with a woman—is one of the oldest human activities. Even now, serving a roast is a symbol of hospitality. Milking, by contrast, did not present the feast-or-famine dilemma; it was a steady business.

Technology plays a big role in the history of milk; every advance in fencing, breeding, and preserving milk made milking more efficient. The result is that consumption of dairy foods is nearly universal in human groups. With the notable exception of East and Southeast Asia, all the European and Middle Eastern cultures, and many Asian and African ones, have a shepherding tradition.

Yogurt, the simplest form of preserved milk, is probably as old as milking itself. Milk "invites its own preservation," writes food maven Harold McGee. Fresh milk curdles quickly, especially in hot weather. Yogurt would have been made—or rather, made itself—simply for lack of refrigeration. The precise origins of yogurt are not known but easy to imagine. When fresh milk is left to stand at room temperature, local bacteria begin to consume the sugars. The milk thickens and becomes tangy with lactic acid. Depending on the bacteria, the result is yogurt, sour cream, or some other cultured milk that stays fresh longer than "sweet" or fresh milk.

Another simple method of preserving nutrients in milk is to remove water. In Iran, milk was reduced to its essence, making a sort of milk bouillon cube to be reconstituted with water. In the thirteenth century, the nomadic Tatar armies of Genghis Khan carried a packed lunch of powdered mare's milk. After skimming off the cream for butter, they dried the skim milk in the sun. Kept in a leather pouch, powdered milk made a convenient meal on the road. It wasn't perishable, and when mixed with water and jostled about on horseback, it made a fermented drink something like yogurt.

Turning milk into cheese is the most sophisticated method of preservation. Gouda, Parmigiano Reggiano, and other traditional aged cheeses mature for two years or longer. Most agree that cheese making is about five thousand years old, but as with yogurt, no one knows exactly where cheese was born, and it's quite possible that shepherds living far apart invented cheese simultaneously. Some of those pioneers were in the French Pyrenees, and in Sumeria, Egypt, five-thousand-year-old pottery bears cheesy residues. Though cheese takes many forms, the basic method—adding rennet to curdle milk—is unchanged, and even particular recipes survive a long time. The recipe for Gaperon, a soft French cheese made with garlic and peppercorns, is twelve hundred years old.

The effects of milk on human diet and culture were widespread and profound. In *About Cows*, Sara Rath says that six-thousand-year-old Sanskrit writings refer to milk as an essential food. The Hindus, who ate and celebrated butter four thousand years ago, honor cows, as did the Sumerians and Babylonians. The Romans, too, were milk drinkers and cheese lovers, and spread the habit throughout Europe. Cattle—in Latin *pecus*, from *pascendum* (put to pasture)—were even used to conduct trades; hence the Roman word for money, *pecunia*. Caesar was evidently irritated to find that Britons in his far-flung empire neglected to grow crops, preferring to live on meat and milk instead.

The Bible makes dozens of references to milk, which represents privilege, wealth, and spiritual blessings, as in "land flowing with milk and honey." Shakespeare's plays are replete with flattering comparisons to milk, butter, and cream, and modern idioms glorify milk. To flatter someone, you *butter him up*; the very best is *la crème de la crème.*

Whether from the human breast or the bovine udder, milk is the universal perfect food—delicious, soothing, nourishing. Milk is delicate, sensuous, transient. It is both simple—a nutritionally complete meal in a glass—and marvelously complex, its various ingredients interacting as if the milk itself were a tiny ecosystem. Indeed, traditional milk is alive, teeming with enzymes and microorganisms that evolved right along with man and woman, usually in the belly.

Milk is diverse. The milks of the ewe and the cow, the mare and the nak, are each different. Even within one species, milk is suggestible: the grass, flowers, and herbs the animal eats create further distinctions, affecting aroma, flavor, and nutrition. The hint of garlic—or more than a hint—in milk is not unknown when animals eat their way through a patch of wild ramps. Gracious and malleable, milk is capable of being transformed into cloud-like whipped cream, silken butter, wobbly yogurt, tangy kefir, creamy *fromage frais*, fluffy ricotta, and dense cheddar.

No wonder this noble food has inspired farmers, chefs, poets—and even politicians. William Cobbett was a member of Parliament, pamphleteer, and reformer who toured the English countryside in the early nineteenth century. A self-appointed defender of farm life and the working man, Cobbett understood peasant life better than most politicians. "When you have a cow," he wrote, "you have it all."

I Reply to the Milk Critics

WE ARE THE ONLY animal to drink milk after weaning and the only animal to drink the milk of another mammal. Whether that's *good* is a hot topic. Some say milk is a cure-all. In the nineteenth century, doctors credited all-milk diets with all manner of therapeutic effects, and even today modern practitioners treat maladies from arthritis to eczema with whole raw milk. The other side says milk is poison.

Robert Cohen is one of milk's fiercest critics. The milk carton on the cover of his book, *Milk: The Deadly Poison*, bears a skull and crossbones, with the ingredients listed in large type: "Powerful growth hormones, cholesterol, fat, allergenic bovine proteins, insecticides, antibiotics, virus, and bacteria." Cohen says dairy foods are linked to acne, allergies, anemia, asthma, constipation, obesity, osteoporosis, and breast cancer. "It is probable," writes Cohen, "that milk consumption is the foundation of heart disease."[10] People for the Ethical Treatment of Animals runs a campaign against milk called *Milk Sucks!* "Dairy products are a health hazard . . . laden with saturated fat and cholesterol. They are contaminated with cow's blood and pus and frequently . . . with pesticides, hormones, and antibiotics."

Press like that could make a vegan out of the most contented milkmaid, and that's exactly what happened to me. I gave up dairy foods to avoid saturated fat and cholesterol and because they were said to be indigestible and allergenic. It was soy milk for me. Later, when I was working with small dairies at the farmers' markets in London, I began to wonder about the bad reputation of milk, cream, butter, and cheese. Our customers were snapping up whole milk and raw milk cheese. As I began to eat real dairy again, it was easy to see why. Soy milk tastes nothing like the real thing. In cooking, butter is irreplaceable. As for cheese, I had barely begun to discover the most complex and diverse form of the remarkably pliable milk.

But I was astounded that people could thrive on the rich dairy foods I thought were indigestible and allergenic. Why weren't butter and cheese lovers plagued with acne, stuffy noses, and stomach cramps? Even more startling, I felt better as I nibbled my way back into real milk, butter, and cheese. Slowly it dawned on me that milk might not be so bad. I began to read more systematically, hoping to uncover the real story of milk—or, more precisely, the whole story. Milk is a complex food, and so are the arguments around it. The critics and the enthusiasts both make good points; the truth about milk seems to fall between the two extreme positions.

What I learned is that all milk is not created equal. Some milk is better than others—for the cow, the environment, and human health. Modern industrial milk is not the same as the milk we used to drink ten thousand years ago—or even one hundred years ago. Not only is traditional milk from cows raised on grass, without synthetic hormones, more delicious than industrial milk from cows raised indoors on corn and soybeans; it's also better for you. Some forms of milk, such as yogurt, are easily digestible—even for people who think they are lactose intolerant. Nutritionally, raw milk has many advantages over pasteurized milk. Now, when people ask, "Is milk is good for you?" I'm likely to answer, "That depends. Which milk?"

The milk critics make three broad charges. They say that milking is inhumane for cows, dairies pollute the environment, and milk is unhealthy. About the first two, they are absolutely right, with one qualification: *industrial* dairies are bad for cows and for the environment, but *traditional* dairy farming is good for both.

According to Jo Robinson, the author of *Pasture Perfect,* when farmers graze dairy cows outside on their natural diet of grass, the cows are happy and healthy. Farmers who switch from confinement dairies and a grain-based diet and let their cows roam outside eating grass watch their vet bills shrink. One reason is that eating grain gives cows the bovine version of acid indigestion, which can lead to stomach ulcers. Large confinement dairies also pollute the environment with stench and manure lagoons. Properly managed grazing, by contrast, enhances soil fertility, water quality, and biodiversity.

The question of health is more complicated. First, the critics contend that humans are not meant to drink the milk of any other species. Second, they say that milk is indigestible for people who don't make enough of the enzyme lactase to digest the sugar lactose. Let's look at each argument.

Is drinking milk unnatural? The critics say that cow milk was "designed" for newborn calves, not for humans. That's true. But this observation does not prove that the human digestive system cannot, or should not, handle milk. After all, the tomato was designed to make more tomato plants, not pasta sauce. In fact, milk and other dairy foods are not only digestible for the vast majority of people—about 85 percent by some estimates—but also highly nutritious. Later, we'll look at important differences between traditional and industrial milk, but for now let's consider its basic components.

Like breast milk, the milk of cows and other mammals is nutritionally complete. All milk is made of the three macronutrients—protein, fat, and carbohydrate—and humans are equipped to digest all three. A good source of complete protein, milk contains all the essential amino acids in the right amounts. Milk contains enough carbohydrates for energy and has a good balance of fats, both saturated and unsaturated.

Because it was made to be the only source of nutrients for growing babies, milk contains everything required to digest and use its nutrients. The fats in milk, for example, enable the body to digest its protein and assimilate its calcium. According to Mary Enig in *Know Your Fats*, the saturated fats in milk (such as butyric acid) are particularly easy to digest because they do not have to be emulsified first by the liver. Unlike polyunsaturated fats, which the body tends to store, the saturated fats in milk are rapidly burned for energy.

Milk is rich in vitamins and minerals. It contains potassium and vitamins C and B, especially B_{12}, which is found only in animal foods. Milk is the major source of the fat-soluble vitamins A and D in the American diet. As Weston Price observed more than seventy years ago, the calcium and phosphorus in milk are particularly important for handsome facial structure and strong teeth. Dairy foods also reduce oral acidity (which causes decay), stimulate saliva, and inhibit plaques and cavities.

GOOD THINGS IN MILK

- Complete protein to build and repair tissues and bones
- Vitamin A for healthy skin, eyes, bones, and teeth
- Vitamin D to aid calcium and phosphorus absorption and for bones and teeth
- Thiamine to help turn carbohydrates into energy and aid appetite and growth
- Riboflavin for healthy skin, eyes, and nerves
- Niacin for growth and development, healthy nerves, and digestion
- Vitamin B_6 to build body tissues, produce antibodies, and prevent heart disease
- Vitamin B_{12} for healthy red blood cells, nerves, and digestion; and to prevent heart disease
- Pantothenic acid to turn carbohydrates and fat into energy
- Folic acid to promote the formation of red blood cells and prevent birth defects and heart disease
- Calcium to make strong bones and teeth; also aids heartbeat, muscle, and nerve function
- Magnesium for strong bones and teeth

- Phosphorus for strong bones and teeth
- Zinc for tissue repair, growth, and fertility

Critics charge that milk is indigestible for people who don't make enough of the enzyme lactase to digest the lactose in milk. This important argument deserves a full discussion. Lactose plays a large role in the history of milk.

The milk sugar lactose is found in no other food—unless you eat yellow forsythia blossoms in the spring. Without the enzyme lactase, drinking milk causes nausea and diarrhea. Raw milk contains lactase, but the enzyme is damaged by pasteurization. Babies, who drink nothing but milk, produce a lot of lactase; this declines steadily until they reach the age of three or four, and then levels off. The logic of this efficiency is clear. Stone Age mothers nursed babies for three or four years. Unless the child drank milk after weaning, lactase production gradually tapered off. The result is that some adults lack sufficient lactase to digest fresh milk easily. The condition is often known as lactose intolerance, but low lactase production is more precise.

Climate explains the evolution of lactase production. Low lactase production is most common in people whose ancestors came from hot climates, such as East and Southeast Asia and parts of Africa. Where fresh milk could not be kept cold, adults never developed the capacity to produce lactase, simply because they didn't drink fresh milk. In colder climates such as northern Europe, however, where fresh milk could be stored for a week or more, people gradually developed the ability to produce lactase as adults. Genetic analysis shows that milk proteins in seventy European cattle breeds evolved along with human genes for lactose tolerance near northern European dairy settlements in the last eight thousand years, a rare example of cultural and genetic coevolution between humans and another species.[11] The genes show that early northern European shepherds were dependent on milk, unlike southern Europeans.

In hot climates, adults with low lactase production didn't forgo dairy foods entirely, however. After all, Italy, Greece, and Israel are but three sunny countries with dairy traditions. Instead they ate cultured or fermented milk products, particularly yogurt, which is easy to digest because it contains little (if any) lactose. Beneficial bacteria have already consumed the lactose and turned it into the lactic acid that imparts the distinctive tangy taste to yogurt. Thanks to these tiny bacteria, almost everyone can digest cultured milk. In cheese making, lactose is also transformed into lactic acid, but more slowly. The longer the cheese has been aged, the less lactose it contains.

This "solution" to the problem of drinking fresh milk was no doubt accidental. Recall that fresh milk left to stand overnight rapidly becomes yogurt with the help of whatever bacteria happen to be about. Quite by chance, shepherds devised many local variations on yogurt—the word is Turkish—including Armenian *matzoon*, Bulgarian *naja,* Egyptian *laban,* Russian *kvass* (a slightly alcoholic yogurt), and Balkan *kefir,* traditionally made with fermented mare milk.

TRADITIONAL VERSUS INDUSTRIAL FOOD PROCESSING

Yogurt and cheese are processed foods. Processed foods have a bad reputation, often justified. But industrial and traditional methods are different: industrial food processing *diminishes* flavor and nutrition, while traditional food processing *enhances* both. When whole wheat is refined into white flour, flavor, fiber, and B vitamins disappear. Cold-pressed olive oil keeps its vitamin E and antioxidants. When grape juice turns into wine, antioxidants form. When cabbage becomes kimchi, the result

> is more vitamin C, enzymes, and good bacteria. Fermented foods like sauerkraut, cheese, and yogurt are among the oldest and most nutritious processed foods. Yogurt is widely associated with longevity.

Traditional cultured milks are not only digestible but also nutritious. According to Harold McGee, beneficial bacteria found in "traditional, spontaneously fermented milks" take up residence in our guts and promote health all over the body. The bacteria secrete antibacterial agents, enhance immunity, break down cholesterol, and reduce carcinogens. The bacteria added to industrial yogurt don't necessarily do the same good work. They're specialized to grow in milk only and can't survive inside the body. Moreover, industrial yogurt may contain only two or three selected microbes, while the traditional version may sport a dozen or more friendly bacteria. "This biological narrowing may affect flavor, consistency, and health value," writes McGee.

Cultured foods are vitally important in traditional diets. In many cultures, yogurt is the only form of milk consumed. When versatile milk is transformed into yogurt and cheese, people all over the world can eat dairy foods—and given how practical, delicious, and nutritious milk is, most do.

Milk is also rich in cholesterol and saturated fat. Does that mean the shepherds and dairy farmers who drink whole milk daily have high cholesterol and heart disease?

Milk, Butter, Cholesterol, and Heart Disease

LET'S RECALL THE GIST of the cholesterol theory of heart disease: eating cholesterol and saturated fat raises blood cholesterol and clogs arteries. If so, the milk critics have a case, because milk is rich in cholesterol and saturated fat. Milk is 87 percent water; the rest is protein, fat, and lactose. An eight-ounce (250 ml) glass of whole milk (typically 3.5 percent fat) contains about 9 grams of fat, most of it saturated—about 66 percent. About 30 percent is monounsaturated, and there's a bit of polyunsaturated fat, too. The typical glass also contains about 35 milligrams of cholesterol, mostly in the fat. (By the way, I never count grams of fat, cholesterol, protein, or anything else—nor do I recommend it—but I offer these figures for complete information.)

This nutritional profile has been enough to indict milk on charges of causing heart disease, but abundant evidence exonerates real milk, butter, and cheese. Many traditional diets include whole milk and butter without adverse effects. In Swiss dairy and Masai shepherd communities, Weston Price found people eating whole milk, cream, and butter to be in excellent health. In the 1960s, long after Price studied the Masai diet, Professor George Mann went to Kenya to test the hypothesis that a diet rich in saturated fat and cholesterol raises blood cholesterol.[12] The Masai are almost pure carnivores, eating mostly milk, blood, and meat. A Masai man drinks up to a gallon of whole milk daily, and on top of that he might also eat a lot of meat containing still more saturated fat and cholesterol. Mann expected the Masai to have high blood cholesterol but was surprised to find it was among the lowest ever measured, about 50 percent lower than that of the average American.

Like the Swiss and Masai diets, the traditional American diet was once rich in whole milk, cream, butter, and meat. At the turn of the last century we ate plenty of butter and other saturated fats. The *Baptist Ladies Cookbook* (1895) and *The Boston Cooking School Cookbook* (1896) include recipes for creamed liver, lamb fried in lard, creamed fish, and oyster pie with a quart of cream and a dozen egg yolks. About 40 percent of the calories in these menus come from fats, with slightly more saturated than unsaturated fats. An English Jewish cookbook in 1846 is similar, but it calls for beef fat instead of lard. These menus would be unremarkable—after all, everyone's grandmother cooked that way—except for one curious, highly relevant fact. In 1900, when these recipes were used and saturated fat was a regular part of the diet, heart disease was rare. The first case of heart disease as we know it was identified by Dr. James B. Herrick in 1912.

In the next hundred years, traditional fats were replaced by industrial fats. The 1931 *Searchlight Recipe Book* reflects the transition in American cooking. This, too, contained recipes with butter and cream, but it also called for vegetable oil and "butter substitute" or margarine. Cooks began to change their recipes, no doubt gradually at first. According to the lipids expert Mary Enig, from 1910 to 1970, butter consumption plummeted from eighteen pounds per person per year to four. During the same period, the percentage of vegetable oils in the diet—including margarine, shortening, and refined oils—soared by 400 percent.

As the table (page 63) shows, from 1935 to 1985, the percentage of saturated fats in the American diet *fell*, while consumption of polyunsaturated vegetable oils more than doubled. (Note, too, that we ate more total fat in 1985, possibly due to larger portions. Not only did the low-fat campaign fail to reduce obesity and heart disease; it simply *failed*.) The changing face of the most popular fats in the diet tells the same story in a different way. In 1890, the main fats we ate were the traditional farm fats: butter, lard, and chicken and beef fat. A hundred years later, the top three fats were polyunsaturated vegetable oils such as soybean and canola oil, rarely found in traditional human diets.

DAILY FAT INTAKE BY TYPE OF FAT, 1930–85

The most dramatic change in the American diet is the increase in polyunsaturated fats, up by 127 percent. The percentage of saturated fats *fell*. Many of the polyunsaturated fats shown are hydrogenated vegetable oils, which raise LDL and reduce HDL.

	1930–35		*1985*	
Type of fat	*Grams*	*%*	*Grams*	*%*
Saturated	59	48	62	38
Monounsaturated	50	40	68	41
Polyunsaturated	15	12	34	21
Total	124	100	164	100

FATS IN THE U.S. FOOD SUPPLY (IN DESCENDING ORDER OF MARKET SHARE)

Note that all the nineteenth-century fats are unrefined with a long history in the human diet. The top three oils in 1990 were unknown in traditional diets.

1890	*1990*
Lard	Soybean oil (70 percent hydrogenated)
Beef fat	Canola oil (often hydrogenated)
Chicken fat	Cottonseed oil
Butter	Peanut oil
Olive oil	Corn oil
Palm oil	Palm oil
Coconut oil	Coconut oil

Source: Mary Enig, *Know Your Fats*.

With this record of fat consumption—fewer saturated fats, more polyunsaturated vegetable oils—proponents of the cholesterol theory would *not* have predicted this: by the 1950s, heart disease was the leading cause of death in the United States. It's a striking fact, worth restating in another way: as consumption of saturated fats *fell* in the first half of the twentieth century, heart disease *rose*. This suggests that something other than butter and other traditional saturated fats is to blame for unhealthy cholesterol and heart disease.

That something is the trans fat in hydrogenated vegetable oils like margarine. As the world now knows, trans fats lower HDL and raise LDL, among other things. Real dairy foods, it appears, are innocent. Back in 1991—when heart doctors were touting vegetable oil spreads—*Nutrition Week* reported that men eating butter ran half the risk of developing heart disease as those eating margarine.[13]

Recent studies cast doubt on the link between dairy foods, high cholesterol, and heart disease. Consider the Finns, who have the highest cholesterol in the world. "According to the [cholesterol theory], this is due to high-fat Finnish food," writes Dr. Uffe Ravnskov, author of *The Cholesterol Myths* and a leading researcher in a group known as the Cholesterol Skeptics. "The answer is not that simple." Within Finland, cholesterol levels vary greatly. In one study, Finns who ate twice as much margarine and half as much butter as other Finns had the *highest* cholesterol. Those with the highest cholesterol also preferred skim milk to whole milk.[14]

WHY I DON'T DRINK SKIM MILK

Let me count the ways. The first reason I don't drink skim milk is flavor—it's in the fat. Second, butterfat helps the body digest the protein, and bones require saturated fats in particular to lay down calcium. Third, the cream contains the vital fat-soluble vitamins A and D. Without vitamin D, less than 10 percent of dietary

> calcium is absorbed.[15] In the American diet, whole milk was the traditional source of vitamins A and D and calcium. Skim milk—especially industrial skim—is an inferior source of both. Skim and 2 percent milk must, by law, be fortified with synthetic vitamin A and synthetic vitamin D_3. There is some evidence that both synthetic vitamins are toxic in excess. Finally, whole milk contains glycosphingolipids, fats that protect against gastrointestinal infection. Children who drink skim milk have diarrhea at rates three to five times higher than children who drink whole milk.[16]

In 2005, researchers reported on a twenty-year study of Welsh men. The high milk drinkers had a lower risk of heart disease than those who drank the least, even though cholesterol and blood pressure were similar in high and low milk drinkers. "The present perception of milk as harmful in increasing cardiovascular risk should be challenged," wrote the authors, "and every effort should be made to restore [milk] to its rightful place in a healthy diet."[17]

As researchers demonstrate every day, many other factors—sugar, lack of B vitamins, too many refined vegetable oils, lack of exercise, smoking—are at work in heart disease. But these anomalies about milk and butter—facts that don't fit the orthodox theory—cry out for explanation.

Meanwhile, I should mention that some studies *have* linked milk consumption and high cholesterol. What could account for that? According to Dr. Kilmer McCully, a student of cholesterol metabolism and the author of *The Heart Revolution*, industrial powdered milk is one culprit. Dried milk powder is created by a process called spray-drying, which creates oxidized or damaged cholesterol. Researchers in 1991 wrote, "Oxidized low-density lipoprotein (LDL) is more atherogenic than native [unoxidized] LDL."[18] In other words, oxidized LDL causes atherosclerosis.

Milk powder containing oxidized cholesterol is a common ingredient in industrial processed foods including milk, yogurt, low-fat cheese, cheese substitutes, infant formula, baked goods, cocoa mixes, and candy bars. Nonfat dried milk is also added to industrial skim and 2 percent milk. In fact, skim milk may be made *entirely* of dried milk powder mixed with water. Unfortunately, the label is misleading. It will simply say "skim milk," not "skim milk powder." The better dairies don't use powdered milk; they make skim milk from whole fresh milk simply by skimming off the cream.

My conclusion that traditional milk is a good thing is not original. In the 1930s and '40s, Dr. Francis Pottenger ran tuberculosis clinics where he treated patients with raw milk from grass-fed cows. A professor at the University of Southern California and president of the American Academy of Applied Nutrition, he published dozens of peer-reviewed articles and founded a hospital for the treatment of asthma. In his day, experts were already blaming milk for high cholesterol, but Pottenger believed traditional milk was falsely accused. In his now classic studies on raw and pasteurized milk, *Pottenger's Cats,* the doctor wrote: "The charge that milk produces high cholesterol in humans is largely based on the premise that the ingestion of cholesterol and the deposit of cholesterol are the same. Extensive use of quality raw milk, cream, and farm eggs with tuberculosis patients failed to produce a single case of hypercholesterolemia [high blood cholesterol] and atheroma [plaque]. A life-time consumption of clean, fresh raw milk from healthy cattle does not produce metabolic diseases. Cholesterol is not the villain; the villain is what man does to his cattle and milk."

I like the way Pottenger put that. As I sorted through the facts about milk and health, it was helpful to keep asking: *which milk?* Many things aren't what they used to be, and milk is one of them.

Traditional and Industrial Milk Are Different

ONE OF MY FAVORITE children's books is Maj Lindman's *Snipp, Snapp, Snurr, and the Buttered Bread,* about Swedish triplets who are hungry for bread and butter. Alas, there is no butter. They go to the family cow, Blossom, who "stood munching her dry hay and looking very sad." When the boys ask nicely for milk with "plenty of cream" so their mother can make butter, Blossom shakes her head sadly; she has none to give. "I know what she needs," says one boy. "Fresh green grass." When spring comes and the pasture turns "green and juicy," they give Blossom a basket of fresh grass. Delighted, she gives back rich cream, and the equally delighted boys have butter for their bread.

First published in the United States in 1934, *The Buttered Bread* is a sweet story, but it's more than that. It nicely illustrates the point—once well known to farmers in Sweden, America, and all over the world—that cows produce the most cream and the best butter when eating lush green pasture, particularly the fast-growing grass of spring and fall. In the Swiss dairy villages Weston Price visited, spring butter was so highly prized it was blessed by priests and used in religious ceremonies. Spring butter from grass-fed cows has been tested in the lab (by Price and others) and found to be superior. Blossom's story is poignant because so few cows today eat fresh grass.

Modern industrial milk and the milk we drank ten thousand years ago—even the milk most Americans (including Great-Aunt Esther in Milford, Illinois) drank fifty years ago—are different. Traditional milk comes from cows fed mostly on fresh grass and hay; it is raw and unhomogenized. Industrial milk comes from cows raised indoors and fed mostly on a corn, grain, and soybean ration, typically with a dose of synthetic hormones to boost milk production. Industrial milk is then pasteurized and homogenized. Real milk is healthier than the industrial kind, and its superior flavor is unmistakable.

Because cows eat grass, traditional milk is seasonal. Ancient shepherds moved animals frequently to fresh pasture for the best grazing. In the winter, the traditional cow was "dry"—pregnant and not producing milk—and in the spring she gave birth to a calf and began giving milk again. Traditional dairy foods naturally reflect this seasonal pattern. In the spring, when fresh pasture for grazing was plentiful, early shepherds had fresh milk, yogurt, and young cheeses. In the winter, when the cows were dry, they ate aged cheeses made the previous summer and fall. The best dairy farmers still raise cows, goats, and sheep on grass—they are known as *grass farmers*—and the better cheese shops offer seasonal cheeses made from the milk of grass-fed animals.

Compared to industrial milk, dairy foods from grass-fed cows contain more omega-3 fats, more vitamin A, and more beta-carotene and other antioxidants. Butter and cream from grass-fed cows are a rare source of the unique and beneficial fat CLA. According to the *Journal of Dairy Science*, the CLA in grass-fed butterfat is 500 percent greater than the butterfat of cows eating a typical dairy ration, which usually contains grain, corn silage, and soybeans.[19]

A polyunsaturated omega-6 fat, CLA prevents heart disease (probably by reducing atherosclerosis), fights cancer, and builds lean muscle. CLA aids weight loss in several ways: by decreasing the amount of fat stored after eating, increasing the rate at which fat cells are broken down, and reducing the number of fat cells. Most studies of CLA and cancer have been conducted on animals, and more research is needed, but findings are encouraging. CLA inhibits growth of human breast cancer cells in vitro. A Finnish team found that women eating dairy from pastured animals had a lower risk of breast cancer than those eating industrial dairy.[20]

The dairy industry is well aware of the commercial opportunity presented by the words *cancer fighting* or *aids weight loss* on milk cartons, and scientists are working on ways to increase CLA in milk without going to the trouble of putting cows on grass. In 2003, the *Journal of Dairy Science* reported that feeding fish oil and sunflower seeds (containing linoleic acid, which cows convert to CLA) raises CLA in milk. There are CLA-fortified milk products in the works, but problems with taste and texture linger. "The addition of CLA to milk decreased overall acceptability, overall flavor, and freshness perception of milk," reported one study coolly.[21] If imitation is the sincerest form of flattery, these "functional foods" or "nutraceuticals," as the industry calls them, pay a high compliment to traditional foods.

Traditional milk is free of synthetic growth hormones. Most industrial milk comes from cows treated with a genetically engineered bovine growth hormone called rBGH (or rBST) to boost milk production. Industrial cows are milked three times a day. Unfortunately for the cow, the hyperproduction stimulated by rBGH increases her risk of mastitis (udder infections) and shortens her life dramatically, from about ten years to five.

Milk from cows treated with rBGH contains higher levels of IGF-1, a naturally occurring growth hormone that is identical in cows and humans. When you drink a glass of milk from a cow treated with rBGH, you get a dose of IGF-1, one of the most powerful of many insulinlike hormones that prompt cells to grow and proliferate. IGF-1 is linked to cancers of the reproductive system, including breast cancer. Because the FDA regards rBGH as safe for human consumption, it does not permit dairy farmers to print "hormone-free" on milk labels, but most dairy farmers who *don't* use hormones find a way to say so. If the label is silent, it's a safe bet the cows were treated with rBGH.

What kind of milk should you buy? Traditional milk is ideal and organic milk second-best. Both are better than industrial milk. Unfortunately, most commercial organic milk comes from cows fed grain, not fresh grass. (All cows must eat some hay for roughage.) Organic cows must have "access" to pasture, but on many large organic dairies, cows spend very little time outside. Grass-fed milk is best, even if it's not organic. Most grass farmers feed cows on grass and hay with a small grain supplement at milking, as I fed Mabel. That's acceptable, because even an ancient wild cow would have eaten some grain from seed heads.

INDUSTRIAL, COMMERCIAL ORGANIC, AND TRADITIONAL MILK

The best choice is traditional milk, but it's not easy to find. Farmers who supply two organic brands, Organic Valley and Natural by Nature, raise cows on pasture. By law, no milk includes antibiotics. If a cow needs antibiotics, her milk is discarded until the drugs have cleared her system.

Type of Milk	*Cows' Diet*	*Cows' Life*	*Synthetic Growth Hormones*	*Pasteur-ized*	*Homo-genized*
Industrial milk	Corn, grain, and soybeans	Stay indoors	Yes	Yes	Yes
Commerical organic milk	Organic corn, grain, and soybeans	Have "access" to pasture	No	Yes	Sometimes
Traditional milk	Mostly grass and hay	Graze outside	No	No	No

Perhaps the greatest difference between traditional and modern milk is pasteurization, routine since the middle of the twentieth century. The French chemist Louis Pasteur invented pasteurization, a form of heat sterilization, in the 1860s to improve the keeping qualities of wine and beer. Gentle pasteurization heats the milk to 145 degrees Fahrenheit for thirty minutes, and standard pasteurization heats it to 161 degrees for fifteen seconds. Ultrapasteurized milk is held under pressure at 280 degrees for two seconds. Milk labeled UHT—ultra high temperature—is ultrapasteurized and then packaged in aseptic boxes sterilized with hydrogen peroxide.

Pasteurization is generally regarded as a sign of progress, a boon for public health—and there is much truth in that. Pasteurization does destroy certain pathogens, including salmonella, *E. coli*, and campylobacter. However, pasteurization also destroys vitamins, useful enzymes, beneficial bacteria, texture, and flavor.

The push for pasteurization in the United States began in the late 1800s and the early 1900s. It was a response to an acute and growing public health crisis, in which infectious diseases like tuberculosis were spread by poor-quality milk. Previously, milk came to the kitchen in buckets from the family cow or in glass jars from a local dairy, but soon, urban dairies sprang up to supply the growing populations in or near cities such as New York, Philadelphia, and Cincinnati.

Owners put the dairies next to whiskey distilleries to feed the confined cows a cheap diet of spent mash called distillery slop. For distribution, the whiskey dairies were efficient: in 1852, three quarters of the milk drunk by the seven hundred thousand residents of New York City came from distillery dairies. The last one in New York City (in Brooklyn) closed in 1930.

The quality of "slop milk," as it was known, was so poor it could not even be made into butter or cheese. Some unscrupulous distillery dairy owners added burned sugar, molasses, chalk, starch, or flour to give body to the thin milk, while others diluted it with water to make more money. Slop milk was inferior because animal nutrition was poor; cows need grass and hay, not warm whiskey mash, which is too acidic for the ruminant belly. Recall from Blossom that cows on fresh grass produce more cream, a measure of milk quality.

Conditions were unhygienic, too. In one contemporary account cited in *The Complete Dairy Foods Cookbook*, distillery cows "soon become diseased; their gums ulcerate, their teeth drop out, and their breath becomes fetid." Cartoons of distillery dairies show morose cows with open sores on their flanks standing or lying in muck in cramped stables. Bovine tuberculosis and brucellosis were common, and cow mortality was high. The people milking the cows were often unsanitary and unhealthy, too. Dairy workers could taint milk with human tuberculosis and other diseases.

A public health crisis was brewing. As distillery dairies became common around 1815, contaminated milk caused fatal outbreaks of diseases including infant diarrhea, scarlet fever, typhoid, tuberculosis, and undulant fever (the human version of brucellosis). Infant mortality, often due to diarrhea and tuberculosis, rose sharply, accounting for nearly half of all deaths in New York City in 1839. Reformers blamed the outbreaks of disease on slop milk. The distillery dairies were like the sausage factories later exposed as dirty and unsafe by Upton Sinclair in his 1906 novel *The Jungle*. Regulation was desperately needed.

Reformers suggested pasteurization to kill pathogens carried in milk. At first, no one suggested that raw milk itself was unsafe, according to Ron Schmid in *The Untold Story of Milk*—merely that milk should be clean. "Demands for pasteurization allowed for the continued production and sale of clean raw milk," writes Schmid, a naturopathic physician. "No one was claiming that all milk should be pasteurized, as even the most zealous proponents of pasteurization recognized that carefully produced raw milk from healthy animals was safe."

This view prevailed, briefly. When a raw milk ban was proposed in New York City in 1907, a coalition of doctors, social workers, and milk distributors defeated it, arguing that safe milk should be guaranteed by inspections, not pasteurization. In 1908, however, a panel of experts appointed by President Theodore Roosevelt concluded that raw milk itself was to blame for food-borne illness. That was the final blow. In 1914, New York required pasteurization of milk for sale in shops. Other states followed suit, and by 1949, pasteurization was the law in most places.

The moral of the tale is clear: the trouble starts when you take a cow away from her natural habitat and healthy diet and force her to become a mere milk machine. By abusing the hapless cow, the distillery dairy owners put human health at risk. Slop milk *was* responsible for thousands of cases of illness and death—most of them preventable by improving cow health and dairy hygiene. But mandatory inspections were not the expedient solution to the crisis; pasteurization was.

Today, thanks to better animal nutrition, hygiene, and widespread testing, the tuberculosis and brucellosis that ravaged nineteenth-century populations (bovine and human) are rare. Yet even now, when slop milk is long gone, pasteurization plays a vital role in the commercial dairy industry. FDA rules say that "raw dairy products shall not be shipped across state lines for direct human consumption." Every day, tankers of raw milk rumble down American highways, but the milk is pasteurized before it's sold to you or me. "For the purpose of current commercial distribution of milk, pasteurization is an undoubted necessity," writes Grohman, a lively advocate for raw milk, in *Keeping a Family Cow*. Why?

The typical dairy farmer pours warm milk into a refrigerated tank after milking. Every few days, a truck goes from dairy to dairy collecting raw milk. Thus the milk of thousands of cows is blended before being shipped to the bottling plant or cheese factory. Pasteurization after collection can prevent contaminated milk from one sick cow, unhygienic dairy worker, or dirty nozzle from tainting the clean milk of dozens of other dairies.

Pasteurization also has practical benefits for the dairy industry: it permits more handling, long-distance shipping, and longer storage. Fresh milk doesn't travel well. Jostling damages its delicate fats and sugars and causes milk to sour. Raw milk lasts about a week, but standard pasteurization extends the shelf life of milk to two or three weeks. Ultrapasteurized milk keeps for eight weeks, and aseptic UHT milk can last ten months without refrigeration.

In practice, pasteurization can have an unsavory effect on hygiene in the dairy. It allows less scrupulous dairy farmers to be lax with cow health and milk handling because they count on pasteurization to destroy pathogens—at least the heat-sensitive ones—that may taint milk. Many dairy insiders believe that dairy inspections, despite the lessons of slop milk, are still inadequate. I've seen some not very clean dairies myself.

Nor does pasteurization guarantee protection against food poisoning. Pathogens such as *Listeria* can survive gentle pasteurization.[22] According to the Ohio State University Extension Service, *Listeria* is slightly more heat-resistant than many other bacteria such as salmonella and *E. coli*, and will grow at temperatures as high as 140 to 150 degrees Fahrenheit. (Recall that gentle pasteurization heats milk to 145 degrees.)

Finally, like any food, both raw and pasteurized milk can carry pathogens. Milk may be contaminated at any point *after* pasteurization—in handling, transportation, storage, or cheese making—just as easily as before. Indeed, the majority of dairy-related food-poisoning cases are traced to pasteurized milk and cheese.

WHY IS FOOD POISONING ON THE MARCH?

Outbreaks of food-borne illness caused by salmonella and other pathogens have risen steadily since pasteurization became standard. The reasons aren't well understood, but salmonella and *E. coli* thrive under the conditions typical in factory farms, including grain feeding, overcrowding, and rapid, mechanized slaughter. Overuse of antibiotics on factory farms has also led to resistance to common antibiotics in strains of salmonella, campylobacter, and *E. coli*. Whatever the cause, the recent advances of these pathogens cannot be blamed on raw milk. When raw milk was the norm, these threats were less common. (For more on a dangerous form of *E. coli* that thrives in grain-fed beef cattle, see page 102.)

Traditional milk differs from industrial milk in one other important way: it is not homogenized. If unhomogenized milk is left to stand overnight, the cream, which is lighter, rises to the top. This is good, because the amount and color of the cream (the yellower, the better) have always been the measure of milk quality, and even today farmers are paid more for more butterfat.

Homogenization forcefully blends the milk and cream, so they never separate. Devised in France around 1900 to emulsify margarine, homogenization pumps milk at high pressure through a fine mesh, reducing its fats to tiny particles. Industrial milk (and even cream) are homogenized during or after pasteurization.

In the United States, homogenization became common soon after pasteurization, largely because it solved two practical problems for the dairy industry. The first was the inconvenient separation of the milk and cream. With pasteurization it was possible to ship milk long distances, but the cream rose in transit, which meant the most valuable part of the milk—the fat—was unevenly distributed from one customer to another. Homogenization spreads the cream throughout the milk, so everyone gets a share. The second problem was cosmetic. After pasteurization, dead white blood cells and bacteria form a sludge that sinks to the bottom of the milk. Homogenization spreads this unsightly mass throughout the milk and makes it disappear.

For many years after its introduction, many Americans declined to buy homogenized milk. "Skeptical consumers were disturbed both by the change in flavor and the absence of the cream line at the top of the bottle," writes Schmid in his milk history. But dairy companies persisted with a campaign to win the public over, and by the 1950s, most milk was homogenized.

Homogenization is entirely unnecessary. It's also ruinous for flavor and texture. It breaks up the delicate fats, producing rancid flavors and causing milk to sour more quickly. According to McGee, it takes twice as long to whip homogenized cream, because the fat particles are smaller and more thickly coated with milk protein. I would only add that unhomogenized whipped cream is noticeably more delicious. The best cheeses, too, are made with unhomogenized milk. Happily, unhomogenized milk is perfectly legal, and a few smaller dairies still sell it, sometimes labeled "cream top" or "cream line." If you find that whole milk with cream on top is too rich to drink straight, just pour off the cream and put it on apple pie.

I Describe the Virtues of Raw Milk

BERNARR MACFADDEN WAS A body builder of the rippling-chest variety you see in old comics. Born in 1868, he was a sickly child but overcame his weak start to become a champion of outdoor activity and fitness. Like many reinvented Americans, he changed his name (choosing a funny spelling) and transformed his body by lifting weights. Macfadden kept fit by walking the twenty-five miles from his house in Nyack to New York City—barefoot. In a long, flamboyant career, he became rich and famous selling exercise equipment and publishing fitness manuals, often using his own splendid physique to illustrate poses akin to Greek statuary. At the age of sixty-five—if pictures don't lie—Macfadden had the sort of body readers of *Men's Health* dream of: a hulking, inverted-pyramid torso atop narrow hips and bulging thighs. Macfadden attributed his fine form to raw milk.

In 1924, Macfadden published *The Miracle of Milk: How to Use the Milk Diet Scientifically at Home*. Having studied nineteenth-century European milk cures, he began to treat people with grass-fed, whole raw milk. He found it useful for a range of conditions from neuralgia to bronchitis to heart disease, but he was particularly enthusiastic about milk's ability to help the scrawny build muscle and the flabby lose fat. He gushes about the "plump cheeks," "firm and shapely breasts," muscle tone, and symmetry of patients who took his milk cure, which involved drinking two to six quarts of raw milk daily.

Raw milk has modern fans, too. A surprising number of commercial dairy farmers prefer it. According to a 1999 survey in *Hoard's Dairyman*, 60 percent of dairy farmers drink raw milk at home. When Schmid, author of *The Untold Story of Milk*, asked dairy farmers why, they told him, it "tastes good" or "makes me feel better" or "I don't like store-bought food." Many dairy farmers tell me the same. Barbara King, who raises Ayrshires in Cayuga County, New York, says, "Raw milk straight from the bulk tank has the best flavor." Another dairyman, a former engineer, told me he's raising ten kids on raw milk. Perhaps they're onto something.

It's no secret that raw milk is more nutritious than pasteurized milk. Pasteurization destroys folic acid and vitamins A, B_6, and C. In 1941, the U.S. government issued a report stating that "the cows of this country produce as much vitamin C as does the entire citrus crop, but most of it is lost as the result of pasteurization." Pasteurization inactivates the enzymes required to absorb the nutrients in milk: lipase (to digest fats); lactase (to digest lactose); and phosphatase (to absorb calcium). Phosphatase explains why raw milk contains more available calcium.[23] Pasteurization also creates oxidized cholesterol, alters milk proteins, and damages omega-3 fats.

Heat destroys or damages lactic acid bacteria in raw milk—the same beneficial bacteria in yogurt that aid digestion and immunity. When left alone in raw milk, the good bacteria kill off harmful bacteria which may taint milk during handling, according to Madeleine Vedel, an American expert on the traditional raw milk cheeses of Provence. When *staphylococcus* is introduced to warm pasteurized milk, it proliferates quickly and dangerously, but when added to warm raw milk, it grows much more slowly and may even be eliminated by good bacteria. "By pasteurizing milk we turn it into the ideal medium for dangerous bacteria," concludes Vedel, who owns the Cuisine et Tradition School of Provençale Cuisine in Arles with her husband, Erick, a French chef.[24]

My friend Joann, the dairy farmer, keeps her arthritis at bay by drinking a cup of raw milk at each milking. The arthritis cure is due to the anti-inflammatory Wulzen factor, identified by the researcher Rosalind Wulzen in raw cream and butter in the 1941 *American Journal of Physiology*. The Wulzen factor also prevents calcification of the joints, hardening of the arteries, and cataracts. Raw butter contains myristoleic acid, a monounsaturated fat that fights pancreatic cancer and arthritis.[25]

THE VIRTUES OF RAW MILK AND CREAM

- Raw milk contains heat-sensitive folic acid and vitamins A, B_6, and C.
- Raw milk contains important heat-sensitive enzymes: lactase to digest lactose; lipase to digest milk fats; phosphatase to absorb calcium, which, in turn, allows for the digestion of lactose.
- Raw milk has beneficial bacteria, including lactic acids, which live in the intestines, aid digestion, boost immunity, and eliminate dangerous bacteria.
- Raw cream contains a cortisonelike agent (the Wulzen factor), which combats arthritis, arteriosclerosis, and cataracts.
- Raw butter contains myristoleic acid, which fights pancreatic cancer and arthritis.

Sources: Thomas Cowan, M.D.; Weston A. Price Foundation; Joann Grohman, *Keeping a Family Cow.*

Dr. Thomas Cowan, a physician in San Francisco, treats many conditions with raw milk, including eczema, diabetes, and arthritis. He is following a long and respectable medical tradition. In the 1920s, the Mayo Foundation, forerunner of the prestigious Mayo Clinic, in Rochester, Minnesota, prescribed an all-milk diet known as "the Milk Cure." In a 1929 article, "Raw Milk Cures Many Diseases," a Mayo doctor described milk as an easily digestible food, rich in enzymes, vitamins, and minerals, with a perfect balance of protein, fat, and carbohydrate. Like Macfadden, the body builder, the Mayo doctors found raw milk effective for weight loss and for many ailments, including poor digestion, inflammation, rheumatism, asthma, skin conditions, bronchitis, high blood pressure, kidney disease, and even heart disease.[26]

Today, in the age of pasteurization, old literature on the benefits of raw milk makes interesting reading. In 1916 and 1917, the *American Journal of Diseases of Children* reported that raw milk prevents scurvy in babies, probably because heat destroys vitamin C. In 1933, the *Ohio Agricultural Experiment Station Bulletin* reported that raw milk promotes growth and calcium absorption. In 1937, the *Lancet* said that children on raw milk had greater resistance to tooth decay and tuberculosis. The Drug and Cosmetic Industry reported in 1938 that certain pathogens do not grow in raw milk but proliferate in pasteurized milk. The good bacteria in raw milk—dubbed *natural antiseptics* by the authors—killed the dangerous ones. Sadly, this science is neglected today.

THE MILK DIET: A MODERN EXPLANATION

Recent studies show that people who consume more milk, yogurt, and cheese lose fat (especially belly fat) and gain lean muscle. It's not clear why. The CLA and omega-3 fats from the milk of grass-fed cows prevent obesity and build lean muscle, but it's likely the subjects in these studies ate industrial dairy foods. In *The Calcium Key,* Professor Michael Zemel, director of the Nutrition Institute at the University of Tennessee, argues that calcium is the secret. Zemel explains how low calcium elevates the hormone calcitriol, which causes the body to hoard calcium and send it to fat cells, where it signals cells to store fat. A calcium-rich diet lowers calcitriol and stimulates weight loss. Zemel found that calcium from dairy foods is strikingly more effective than calcium from fortified foods or supplements.[27] Whole raw milk is the best source of calcium; the body needs the enzyme phosphatase (destroyed by heat) and vitamins D (in the fat) to absorb calcium.

Is raw milk safe? Like vegetables or meat, milk can be contaminated with pathogens, but raw milk is not inherently more susceptible than pasteurized milk or any other food. Clean raw milk from a healthy cow, carefully handled by a conscientious farmer, is safe. Hygiene starts in the dairy. Crowded, poorly fed, and weak herds are more susceptible to disease. As we've seen, the cow's ideal habitat is outdoors and her best diet is grass. During milking and handling, the careful farmer avoids contamination from pathogens by using clean buckets, strainers, and other equipment. Milk must be rapidly chilled after milking and kept cold.

I grew up on raw milk, neglected it for years, and now go to some trouble to get it. If you fancy raw milk, find a sparkling clean dairy—ideally one you can visit—with healthy, grass-fed cows and a farmer who drinks raw milk. The best choice is a certified dairy, where the cows are regularly tested for tuberculosis and brucellosis. State law on raw milk sales varies widely, but in about two thirds of the states it is possible to buy raw milk legally in some fashion. California, Connecticut, and New Mexico permit certified raw milk in shops. In many states, including New York, raw milk may be sold at certified farms. Others allow raw milk to be sold as pet food (nod, wink). Some dairy farmers sell a "cow share," which entitles you to a few gallons of milk each week.

One caution: some traditional foods, like sauerkraut and wine, keep well and improve with age. Raw milk is not one of them. Fresh milk must be consumed—or made into yogurt or cheese—in a week or so. Aseptic UHT milk and other foods engineered to last forever have clear commercial advantages, but they come at the price of lost flavor and nutrients. Remember this rule of thumb: *eat foods that spoil—but eat them before they do.*

Fortunately, shepherds long before us spent many hours perfecting a way to preserve perishable raw milk for a rainy day—or more precisely, for a long, cold winter. From fresh spring milk, they made cheese. Traditional pressed cheeses can mature for as long as ten years. The dense, butterscotch flavor of an aged Gouda, the crunch of a two-year-old Parmigiano Reggiano, the melting saltiness of a cave-aged Gruyère—these are the treasures of raw milk transformed. "Cheese," said the editor and critic Clifton Fadiman, is "milk's leap toward immortality."

I Learn to Appreciate Proper Cheese

WHEN I WAS LITTLE, the only thing I knew about cheese was that we didn't approve of the rubbery, individually wrapped slices I spied in the lunch boxes of other kids—that was not real cheese. We did buy undyed cheddar for grilled cheese sandwiches, but other than that, my ignorance was total. When I was about ten, we visited our friends Alan and Karen Furst on Bainbridge Island, and I was riveted when Karen grated a hunk of Parmesan over pasta. I had only seen it already grated, in jars.

Today I do grate Parmigiano Reggiano, but a cheese course after dinner is usually beyond my appetite. Most of my friends are more experienced eaters than I am—with all foods, except, perhaps, tomatoes—and some, like Robin, who has a place in Provence—really know cheese. You can't be interested in raw milk or the butterfat in Jersey milk, as I am, without getting to know cheese lovers. Turophiles—from the Greek *tyros* for cheese—are genial types, and some of their enthusiasm has rubbed off on me. I can almost find my way around a cheese counter, and now and then I'll even do my own little tastings, comparing, say, a couple of salty pecorinos on Robin's zucchini carpaccio.

If there is one obsession in the cheese world, it is—rightly I think—with the milk itself, from which all good cheese is born. The cheese is only as good as the milk, and if there is one mark of distinction for cheese, it is being made from raw milk. Like wine drinkers, cheese lovers do make other distinctions—about history, method, *terroir*. They're notably respectful of tradition ("Charlemagne's favorite cheese"). They talk dreamily of cows all but hand-fed a particular mix of herbs and grasses on a certain slope in a certain Swiss village at a certain time of the year. They swoon over the inspired cheese maker who gently bathes washed-rind cheese in the local apple brandy.

But raw milk is the hottest topic, and with good reason. Raw milk is important to cheese. The enzymes and beneficial bacteria in raw milk aid fermentation. Pasteurized milk limits the action of rennet and retards ripening. Though many good cheeses are made from pasteurized milk, cheeses made from raw milk often contain more complex, subtle flavors—sometimes richer, sometimes mellower. People also swear by raw milk cheese for its beneficial enzymes and bacteria, which are tonics for digestion and immunity.

Many of the best American farmstead cheeses—cheeses made from the milk of the farm's own herd—are made with raw milk, and in the better cheese shops, more than half the cheese for sale are, too. "Pasteurization destroys the natural enzymes essential to the production of aromatic compounds and kills the bacteria responsible for complexity," says Rob Kaufelt, the proprietor of Murray's Cheese Shop in New York City. "Flavor in cheese is related to complexity, and those with a passion for cheese love complexity."

FLORAL MILK AND HERBAL CHEESE

The diversity in well-managed pasture brings a vast array of aroma and flavor to milk and cheese. According to the cheese magazine *Caseus*, aromatic elements in milk called *terpenes*—the organic compounds in essential

> oils—can be traced to particular plants. For example, an increase from 11 to 35 percent of sweet woodruff in a cow's diet produces from 32 to 42 percent increase of a specific terpene in milk. Dovefoot geranium and orchard grass have a similar effect. Aromas vary by season, too. In the winter, grasses dominate and the aromas are less varied and intense. Come summer, weeds and herbs such as yellow bedstraw, common chicory, thyme, mint, and yarrow add measurably to aromas. In southern Italy—as on good pasture anywhere—meadows can contain more than seventy species. Says the writer Italo Calvino, "Behind every cheese there is a different pasture of a different green under a different sky."

For about four thousand years, all cheese was made with raw milk, the only milk there was. But in the age of industrial milk and cheese, raw milk cheese has come under the same cloud of suspicion as raw milk itself. In the United States, the law concerning raw milk cheese hasn't changed since 1949. Cheese makers must either use pasteurized milk or age their cheese for at least sixty days, beyond which time, presumably, all the deadly pathogens have given up. Young—or fresh—cheeses such as chèvre, mozzarella, and ricotta must be made with pasteurized milk. The French, naturally, think that's foolish, and eat young raw milk chèvre and Brie with impunity.

In the United States, the sixty-day rule applies to American as well as imported cheeses. That means that if you see a wheel of young raw milk Brie in an American shop, it is contraband. Fans of raw milk cheese love contraband. They are in the habit of bringing young raw milk cheeses home from Europe, palms sweaty as they try to conceal the aroma emanating from their suitcases at customs. Now and then cheesemongers succumb to the same impulse. In the cheekier shops, you might see a sign along these lines: GET THIS CHEESE BEFORE THE FDA GETS US. Good idea.

> **NOT QUITE RAW**
>
> One very gentle method of pasteurization is of particular interest to turophiles: thermalization. The International Dairy Federation defines it as heating milk to 145 to 150 degrees Fahrenheit under "flowing" conditions—rather than in a vat—for fifteen to twenty seconds. Certain bacteria (good and bad) are destroyed, but some enzymes are left unharmed, which leads to better flavor in cheese. Several European cheeses—Berthaut Epoisses, a blue called Persillé du Beaujolais, and Il Fortetto, a pecorino—are made with thermalized milk. The import rules around thermalized cheese are murky, but they're usually regarded as raw milk cheeses under U.S. law.

The bureaucrats are mistaken. Raw milk cheese is very safe. The beneficial bacteria created by fermentation actually inhibit the pathogens everyone is so worried about. The acidity of cheese (a pH of four to five) kills harmful bacteria. Nor does pasteurization guarantee safety. Nearly all outbreaks of food poisoning from milk and cheese in recent decades involved pasteurized milk. A review of foodborne illnesses from 1973 to 1992 in the *Journal of Food Protection* found no outbreaks attributed to raw milk cheese aged more than sixty days.

Catherine Donnelly, a professor at the University of Vermont, also concluded that pasteurization does not ensure the safety of aged cheese and may, in fact, *reduce* safety. Donnelly found that raw milk itself is seldom, if ever, to blame when cheese contains pathogens such as campylobacter. Typically, contamination is the result of unsanitary or ill workers or poor cheese-making methods, such as too little salt or acidity. "Unpasteurized milk used in some cheeses (such as Swiss and Parmesan) may even retard the growth of pathogens in aged cheese," writes Donnelly.

Nevertheless, from time to time officials—citing food safety—drop hints about outlawing raw milk cheese altogether. A ban on raw milk cheese would mean the end of classic European cheeses such as Roquefort, Parmigiano Reggiano, Gruyère, Manchego, Montgomery cheddar, and American cheeses such as Thistle Hill Tarentaise, made in North Pomfret, Vermont, from grass-fed, raw Jersey milk—a bleak prospect.

At the mere suggestion of regulatory threats to traditional cheese making, however, artisan and farmstead cheese makers, cheesemongers, and cheese lovers rally. Gerd Stern, a past president of the American Cheese Society, says there is no scientific evidence to support claims that raw milk cheese is dangerous. In a very American way, Stern regards using raw milk as a question of liberty, not only for cheese lovers but also for cheese makers. "Unique microclimates and traditional variegated pastures with many wild flowers and herbs—rather than single-crop grass—give a rich variety of herbal and floral flavors to raw milk," he says. "We believe cheese makers should have the right to use it."

3

Real Meat

Why Even Vegetable Farms Need Animals

HISTORICALLY, FARMING WAS always an uncertain proposition, with the constant risk of uneven harvests due to droughts, floods, and locusts. But in the 1940s and '50s, the second-oldest profession became much more predictable. Farmers achieved more reliable crops and vastly bigger yields with three key technologies: chemicals, laborsaving equipment, and breeding. Genetic experts designed highly productive, disease-resistant plants and animals, from corn to beef cattle, which mature quickly and efficiently. With these new methods, farms overflowed with cheap food.

Conjuring up images of bursting grain silos to feed the world's hungry, the masters of this technological boom called it the Green Revolution. It's a flattering moniker, but misleading, because the side effects were nasty. Chemicals employed to achieve huge yields included powerful pesticides, nitrogen fertilizers derived from World War II bombs, synthetic growth hormones, and antibiotics. Like traditional factories belching out smoke, factory farms also produce unsavory waste: noxious manure lagoons, pesticide drift, and nitrogen runoff polluting rivers and streams. It was as if the methods of the Industrial Revolution had been applied to farming.

Before long, the Industrial Farming Revolution begat a counter-revolution. In my view, this was a truly green revolution—environmentally sound, humane, and healthy. In the 1970s, food co-ops and health food shops in Berkeley, California, started selling organic and whole foods, and chefs like Alice Waters at Chez Panisse and Nora Pouillon in Washington, D.C., started to buy local and seasonal foods. Small farmers like us, using ecological methods, began to sell directly to a newly conscious public at farm stands and farmers' markets.

At first, this new market was mostly for fruits and vegetables. Although some farmers (like my family) kept a cow or chickens for home use, most of us were growing fruit, vegetables, herbs, and flowers for local markets and chefs—not meat and dairy. That was partly because processing, transporting, and selling foods such as beef and butter is more costly and complicated than taking cucumbers to market.

But there were also cultural reasons, I think, for the emphasis on produce. In the early 1970s, vegetarians claimed the nutritional and environmental high ground. As my friend Joann wrote in 1990, "So vigorously has the vegetarian movement pursued the twin themes of whole food and rejection of animal products that in the minds of most people, to be committed to whole foods or organic gardening without being a vegetarian takes some explaining."

Fans of organic and local foods have sometimes been outright hostile to meat. In 1982, we started a farmers' market in Takoma Park, Maryland, and it soon grew popular. When we invited Forrest Pritchard, a young Virginia beef farmer, to the farmers' market in 2001, a few customers objected—loudly. Letters to the editor were heated. The farmers' market was for vegetarians, they protested. (Er . . . we thought it was for *farmers*.) But times change. Today Forrest does a brisk trade in grass-fed beef and pastured poultry, and in 2004, members of the Takoma Park food co-op, after an emotional debate, voted to start selling natural meat.

No one—vegetarian or omnivore—who cares about farming, nutrition, or ecology can afford to ignore animals. Animal products account for the majority (51 percent) of American agriculture, about one hundred billion dollars in annual farm sales. The average American eats 186 pounds of meat annually, including beef, poultry, lamb, pork, and veal, and almost 600 pounds of milk, cheese, and ice cream. Unfortunately, most of these foods are produced on large industrial farms with methods that degrade the environment and diminish nutrition. The question is not whether one should be able to buy meat at farmers' markets, but what *kind* of meat.

Today many farmers like Forrest raise animals with humane and ecological methods for local and national markets. Farmers' markets, food co-ops, and specialty shops sell beef, lamb, pork, game, poultry, eggs, milk, butter, and cheese to go with the seasonal produce. In supermarkets and casual restaurant chains, Niman Ranch represents five hundred independent family farms raising beef, pork, and lamb the traditional way. In the market for organic foods, demand for meat and dairy is growing fastest.

Not long ago, the food world was splintered. There were vegetarians and meat lovers, gourmands and environmentalists. Often they had little in common, but today we all rally around slow and local foods—*slocal* foods, as I call them. (Slow Food is the very American name of a group born in Italy as a protest against fast food. Dedicated to traditional foods, Slow Food has chapters all over the world.) Today, vegetarians who learned about heirloom tomatoes twenty years ago are discovering raw milk cheese, health-conscious people are asking how pastured eggs have more omega-3 fats than industrial eggs, and steak lovers are listening to animal rights advocates who decry factory farms.

As I pondered this cultural shift, I discovered something curious about animals. Every ecological farm—even a vegetable farm—needs them. When I was little, it never occurred to me that we imported horse manure from local stables for soil fertility. Our own cow and chickens simply left their manure on pasture; we didn't compost it for the zucchini. Much later, I learned that the ideal farm builds soil fertility from its own resources—a bedrock principle of organic and biodynamic farming.

The mixed farm is best. In addition to fertilizer, animals provide meat, milk, and eggs, and—amazingly—require very little in return. Broadly speaking, there are two kinds of animals—grazers and omnivores—and each has its place on the farm. Grazers, such as cattle, sheep, and goats, live on grass and other vegetation. With four stomachs, a special system of fermentation, and help from beneficial bacteria, ruminants convert forage that is literally indigestible to humans (grass is mostly cellulose) into high-quality fat and protein. Ruminants work this magic even on marginal land, where the soil is poor or cannot be tilled because it is hilly, rocky, or marshy.

Omnivores such as pigs and chickens can also convert plants to protein and fat, but they need more nutrients—namely, complete protein—than pasture has. Along with grass, they eat kitchen scraps, field stubble, and wild foods. The adaptable pig will eat almost anything, from acorns to whey to coconut. Poultry, too, are clean-up animals, eating grain, grass, insects, worms, and leftovers including eggshells and sour milk.

On ecological farms, animals also provide labor. By labor, I don't mean animals trained to serve, such as border collies herding sheep or draft horses at the plow, but when animals intended for market—that is, to be eaten—do useful farmwork. Pigs, for example, like to root; they clear brush and trees like bulldozers. They will snuffle happily for corn the farmer buries in cattle bedding, and, as they forage, the pigs aerate the straw and manure, creating rich compost. Cattle improve poor pastures by grazing, which increases plant diversity, and goats will clean up a thorny hedgerow. Geese and turkeys roaming a vineyard keep weeds down, eat insect pests, and build soil fertility with manure—three economic benefits to the farmer before she so much as collects an egg, sells a turkey breast, or bottles the wine.

Fertilizer, weed and pest control, improving pasture, turning whey and old sweet corn into bacon and eggs—these are some of the virtues of keeping animals. Even if the farmer never slaughters her cow or chickens, they will work without instruction or complaint—grazing and pecking are instincts, after all—*and* there will be butter and eggs for the vegetarians. Animals even benefit the farm ledger. Farmers who raise cows and chickens on pasture save money on feed, fertilizer, and vet bills.

It's too bad that industrial agriculture has no use for the traditional role of animals. When hyperproduction became the chief goal of agriculture, we took animals off lush rolling fields and into dark and crowded factories, stuffing them on grain sprayed with chemicals. As we'll see, the consequences for animal health and happiness, the environment, and the quality of the meat, poultry, and eggs we eat are unhappy, indeed.

How Factory Farms Wreck the Natural Order

DOWN ON THE FACTORY FARM, the idea is to bring animals to market weight quickly and cheaply. To that end, traditional animal husbandry has been replaced by industrial methods: cheap, often unnatural food, fattening diets, antibiotics, steroids. The less space for animals to move around, the better; exercise wastes precious feed calories, and that costs money. Whether the farmer keeps cattle, pigs, or poultry, the motto on industrial farms is the same: sit down, shut up, and eat.

Fans of the species *Bos taurus* make the enthusiastic, but not unreasonable, claim that cows changed the world. "The history of what we think of as civilization is, with very few exceptions, a story intertwined with cattle, a narrative pulled along by oxen, a growth nurtured with butter and cheese," writes M. R. Montgomery in *A Cow's Life*. Whether raised for labor, milk, or meat, the genus *Bos* shares a long history with humankind. From the aurochs to the Aberdeen Angus, many *Bos* species have made themselves useful and (not by accident) have also been successful at spreading progeny. Except for small pockets—above the Arctic Circle, some tropical spots—*Bos* covers the globe.

This comes as no surprise because keeping cattle is easy. All a ruminant needs is grass. From Ireland to Argentina to New Zealand, cattle are traditionally raised on pasture, and until recently U.S. cattle were raised chiefly on grass and hay, too. In the 1950s, however, beef farming changed sharply, thanks to a surplus of cheap corn and soybeans. Ranchers saw that cattle gained weight faster on grain, and unlike grass, grain is available all year. Today most industrial cattle are fattened on grain—a dramatic change in evolutionary terms.[1]

With more marbling (intramuscular fat) than grass-fed beef, "corn-fed" beef was promoted as tender and soon regarded as superior. Grass-fed beef is as lean as a skinless chicken breast, while feedlot cattle are about 30 percent fat by weight—technically obese. Indeed that's the goal. To win the label USDA Prime, beef needs a certain amount of intramuscular fat between the twelfth and thirteenth ribs. To achieve this, a steer must wear a layer of fat, an inch or more deep, beneath the skin. Later, this excess fat is usually trimmed away by butchers and cooks in search of the lean meat we demand. We've made cattle too fat for our own taste.

The new grain diet had unforeseen consequences. Grains give cattle an acid stomach. When calves are weaned and begin eating grain instead of grass, they become ill. The more acid gut of grain-fed cattle increases the risk of illness from *E. coli* in people. Finally, grain-fed beef is less nutritious than grass-fed beef, which has more omega-3 fats, vitamin E, and beta-carotene.

The insults to beef cattle don't stop there. To prevent illness and speed weight gain, industrial cattle are fed antibiotics. Antibiotic use in farm animals has increased ten- or twentyfold since the 1950s.[2] Overuse of antibiotics leads to drug resistance. For farmers, that means using ever-stronger drugs to fight pathogens. For doctors, it means that common antibiotics no longer work on human patients. The Campaign to End Antibiotics Overuse says that "antibiotic resistance is reaching crisis proportions, resulting in infections that are difficult, or impossible, to treat." The American Medical Association opposes the use of human antibiotics for nontherapeutic use in animal farming, and the European Union bans human antibiotics in animals as growth promoters.

Industrial cattle are treated with growth hormones (also called steroids) to fatten them faster. The natural hormones estradiol, progesterone, and testosterone and synthetic hormones zeranol and trenbolone acetate are typically implanted in the ear. Environmental estrogens (as opposed to those made in the body) are called endocrine disruptors because they alter the body's natural hormonal balance. Excess estrogen is linked to reproductive cancers including breast, prostate, and testicular cancer, and since 1950, such cancers have risen sharply. Breast cancer is up 55 percent, testicular cancer up 120 percent, and prostate cancer up 230 percent. According to Dr. Samuel Epstein, a professor of environmental medicine at the University of Illinois School of Public Health and the founder of the Cancer Prevention Coalition, "the risk of breast and other cancers only increases with the uncontrolled use of hormones in meat."

A grave risk from eating industrial beef is mad cow disease, or bovine spongiform encephalopathy. Again the culprit may be what factory farmers force these herbivores to eat. In addition to grain, cattle may be fed less wholesome things: rendered poultry and pork, chicken litter containing feathers and manure, and—most disturbing—parts of other cattle unfit for humans.

Turning cattle into carnivores and cannibals could prove ruinous. In Britain, where mad cow disease devastated the beef industry, cattle probably contracted BSE from eating infected cattle or sheep with scrapie, the ovine version of the disease. Mad cow disease, which appears in similar form in many species including deer and cats, is caused by deformed proteins that leave spongy holes in the brain. The result is drooling, dementia, paralysis, and death. The rare human version, called variant Creutzfeldt-Jakob disease, is similarly grisly and always fatal.

In 1997, the United States banned the feeding of cattle meat and bone meal—the parts most likely to carry BSE—to other cattle. Only two months before the first U.S. case of BSE surfaced in 2003, the FDA reported three hundred violations of the feed ban and the General Accounting Office estimated many more. Even if it were perfectly enforced, the feed rule—like the brain of a mad cow victim—is full of holes. In 2005, bovine fat and blood were still permitted, along with restaurant leftovers, or "plate waste," which means cattle eat the beef with broccoli someone didn't finish. Ground-up pigs and chickens were also still permitted as cattle feed. Because pigs and poultry are themselves fed cattle parts, that means infected cattle matter can end up in cattle feed. In Britain, BSE was brought under control only after a total ban on feeding mammals to cattle.

No one knows how many American cattle have BSE, but many observers fear it is already common. Japan tests every market-bound animal for BSE, and Britain tests every animal older than twenty-four months. In 2005, the United States tested thirty-seven thousand of thirty-seven million cattle slaughtered: 1 percent.[3] If mad cow disease worries you, choose grass-fed, organic, or biodynamic beef.

Humans have been raising pigs for at least ten thousand years and hunting wild boar for much longer. Despite being shunned by two great religions, pork is the world's most popular meat. The pig has the distinction of being the only mammal whose skin we eat. "Who can resist the crackling from roast pork?" asks the food writer Anne Dolamore.[4]

Crackling! The word is sure to make southerners wistful about Grandma's Sunday dinners. Perhaps more than any other animal, the pig is associated with its fat. Irish legend tells that Saint Martin created the pig from a piece of fat, and lard is traditional in many cuisines, from Europe to China to Indonesia. On the island of Borneo, pork, lard, and rice make up the typical dinner, and the fat of wild boar—only its fat, not lean meat—is considered the unique source of physical, sexual, and spiritual vitality. In nineteenth-century America, lard was the fat of choice for frying and baking. Well into the twentieth century, "lard ruled the kitchen and the palate," says the culinary historian Bruce Kraig.[5] Unlike other animal fats, lard makes a dish on its own. A Tuscan specialty, *lardo*, is nothing more than a ribbon-thin square of lard, cured with salt and rosemary.

That people love pork is no mystery—it's delicious. Pigs are popular with farmers, too: they eat anything, fatten easily, breed quickly, and work hard. Indeed most farms have more pig labor than pig tasks, and the working pig is happy rummaging through forests, old orchards, and hedgerows.

Sadly, this is not the picture of pigs on factory farms. Raised indoors in crowded pens, they cannot pursue their natural impulse to root. Concrete or slatted floors allow for easy removal of manure, but they also cause arthritis and deformed feet. Factory pigs are deficient in vitamin E and selenium, antioxidants found in pasture.[6] Confined pigs are subject to infections, including a fatal form of gastroenteritis; to stave off illness, farmers feed them antibiotics. A strain of salmonella found in swine is resistant to an important antibiotic, fluoroquinolone.[7] (Growth hormones may not be used in pigs.)

Under the stress of crowded conditions, pigs bite each other's tails and cause infections. To preempt tail biting, factory farmers snip off the tails with wire cutters (without anesthetic), leaving a hypersensitive stump which pigs work to keep away from the teeth of other pigs. This is called *avoidance behavior*. That's the theory, anyway, but a British study in 2003 found that tail docking *increases* tail biting.[8]

A happy chicken is up with the dawn, lays an egg in the late morning, and when the farmer opens the little chicken house door, she heads outside to hunt for insects in the grass. The occasional dust bath—rolling around in dry soil, fluffing the dust under her feathers—keeps her free of pests. At dusk, the hen goes inside on her own, safe from predators, to her dinner of grain and oyster shell. That's how our chickens live at the farm. Their contented cooing as they settle for the night is one of my favorite sounds.

Not long ago I was in a battery chicken house. It is not a memory likely to fade quickly. Dark and dusty, the barn smelled of ammonia—the sharp, unmistakable odor of uncomposted chicken manure. Stacked in long rows, the wire cages were shorter than my arm and half as deep. Three hens cowered in each cage, with no room to move around. "These cages were built for *nine* hens," said the farmer, with some pride.

Because they never see the light of day, factory hens lose the natural rhythm essential to egg laying. Instead of sunlight, artificial lights tell their bodies when to lay eggs. With no room to move, nest, or forage, a hen has nothing to do but eat, drink, and drop an egg through the wire on a narrow tray or conveyor belt.

Chickens require complete protein, and a good source is insects, grubs, and worms. Factory chicken feed often includes protein from less savory sources: poultry parts and feathers, rendered cats and dogs, beef fat, and cattle bone meal. In crowded battery egg operations, pathogens thrive. Salmonella can make its way into factory eggs, usually via cracked shells, but occasionally before being laid. If the flock is known to be infected, eggs go to the "breakers" market rather than being sold whole. Breakers are pasteurized and made into liquid egg products for restaurants.

Chickens raised for meat—broilers—are also crammed in dark barns. A typical factory chicken barn is eighteen thousand square feet with twenty to forty thousand birds. At the lower density of twenty thousand birds, that's less than one square foot per bird. Crowded like this, chickens become aggressive and peck each other, so farmers cut their beaks off when they're chicks. Birds are confined and the temperature is kept warm because exercise and generating body heat burn calories, and speedy weight gain is the goal.

To combat rampant campylobacter, salmonella, and *E. coli*, farmers feed broilers antibiotics like fluoroquinolone, with now familiar effects on antibiotic resistance. Strains of *E. coli* and salmonella no longer respond to tetracycline, and some campylobacter bacteria are resistant to Cipro, the antibiotic of choice for foodborne illness. In 1989, researchers showed that more antibiotic-resistant strains are found in confinement hens than in free-range birds.[9] In 2000, the FDA proposed to ban fluoroquinolone for use on poultry, but the effort has been stalled by drug companies. Meanwhile, two large chicken producers (Tyson and Perdue) stopped using fluoroquinolone voluntarily. If a bird does happen to carry pathogens, the meat can be contaminated (usually from stray fecal matter) on high-speed evisceration lines. Industrial agriculture, of course, has the answer: your chicken breast is bleached with chlorine.

FACTORY CHICKEN AND CAMPYLOBACTER

Researchers tested four chicken brands—two conventional (Tyson, Perdue) and two antibiotic-free (Bell & Evans, Eberly)—for strains of campylobacter resistant to the antibiotic fluoroquinolone. Tyson and Perdue had stopped using fluoroquinolone a year before the test, showing that strains persist.

% of Chickens Carrying Drug-Resistant Campylobacter Bacteria

Tyson	96
Perdue	43
Bell & Evans	13
Eberly	5

Source: Johns Hopkins Bloomberg School of Public Health, 2005.

Apologists for industrial farming repeat one argument like a mantra: this food is cheap, and people want it that way. But the real costs are seldom reckoned. According to *Environmental Health Perspectives*, "Industrial agriculture depends on expensive inputs from off the farm . . . many of which generate wastes that harm the environment; it uses large quantities of nonrenewable fossil fuels; and it tends toward concentration of production, driving out small producers and undermining rural communities."[10]

Small and independent farms are disappearing. The beef, pork, and poultry industries, once made up of thousands of family farms, are increasingly concentrated. In Iowa, the number of hog farms dropped from 64,500 in 1980 to 10,500 in 2000, while the number of hogs—about 15 million—stayed level. Cornell University says that New York State will lose 6,000 dairy farms in the next fifteen years.

When counted honestly, the financial costs of industrial agriculture mount quickly. Every American foots the bill to clean up water polluted by manure lagoons. The EPA says that waste water from farms contains nitrogen, pathogens, heavy metals, hormones, and antibiotics. Excess nitrogen has created a "dead zone" in the Gulf of Mexico the size of New Jersey. Eighty percent of the American grain crop, which requires heavy doses of nitrogen and pesticides, is fed to livestock, even though they could be eating grass. Industrial cattle eat corn, wheat, soy, and cottonseed oil because this feed is subsidized. From 1995 to 2004, taxpayers spent ninety-one billion dollars on these four crops alone.

The dismaying fact is that industrial farming is a net loss. As Richard Manning writes in *Against the Grain*, in 1940, the average American farm used one calorie in fossil fuels to raise 2.3 calories of food. By 1974 (the most recent figures available), the ratio was 1:1, *before* adding the cost of processing food or transportation. Today a farmer spends thirty-five calories in fossil fuels to produce just one calorie of feedlot beef and sixty-eight calories for a calorie of pork.

No, Virginia—this food ain't cheap.

Why Grass Is Best (and I Don't Mean for Tennis)

All flesh is grass.
—Isaiah

JOEL SALATIN IS AN irrepressible evangelist for traditional animal husbandry. Salatin believes the assembly-line logic of industrial agriculture has turned farmers from independent yeomen into "serfs," slaving for food industry masters to produce cheap food, fast. A strapping man with charisma to spare, Salatin surprises no one when he rejects the role of serf. He prefers to raise beef, poultry, and eggs as God intended. An enthusiastic Christian, capitalist, libertarian, and environmentalist, he likes to count former vegetarians among his customers. When I'm on his farm, or at a farmers' market where I can buy his meat, I'm one of them.

A born sloganeer, Salatin calls his product *salad bar beef.* He knows the term makes you do a double take. It's the cattle, of course, who eat at the salad bar, a mix of fescue, orchard grass, red clover, bluegrass—whatever grows in Swoope, Virginia. Salatin's definition of *salad bar beef*, however, goes well beyond grazing. Salad bar beef is never fed any grain, corn, soybeans, antibiotics, or hormones. It's lean, tender, and tasty—never bland or gamey. It's nutritionally superior to beef fattened on grain, with more omega-3 fats, beta-carotene, and vitamin E. It's seasonal, too. Industrial beef is bred year-round, but on Salatin's farm, calves are born in late spring, amid the dandelions, as he likes to say—never in icy January.

Last but not least, salad bar beef is slaughtered, butchered, and sold locally. Even when food lovers in far-off cities call the farm to order meat, having read about Salatin's farm in *Gourmet* or the *New York Times*, he refuses to ship his food. Salatin is a purist, to be sure. Fine—the world needs purists. If everyone raised salad bar beef, Salatin says, "City folks could enjoy beef without a guilty conscience."

Farmers who raise animals on pasture (being modest types) call themselves grass farmers, because "all they do" is grow grass. The method is ingeniously simple: instead of taking feed to animals, grass farmers let animals go to the feed. The most nutritious pasture is fast-growing, adolescent grass. When the animals have trimmed the best of the new growth, farmers move them to fresh pasture. It's called rotational grazing, and it works, says one farmer, because "grass doesn't like to walk around, and cows do."

Nature is their inspiration. Wild herbivores like zebras travel in herds and move frequently for fresh forage, leaving yesterday's manure behind—just what grass farmers do with animals. In the wild, flocks of birds follow the zebras, while grass farmers send poultry in after livestock. As the grass recovers from being grazed by ruminants, poultry scratch at cow pats and aerate the manure (so it decomposes) while they grow fat or lay eggs eating protein-rich fly larvae.

Grass farming is profitable. Farmers save on labor, repairs, fuel, oil, seed, fertilizer, pesticides, and vet bills. Grazing makes use of marginal land and produces excellent yields, directly related to pasture health and how often animals move. Cattle digestion is complex, but this general rule applies: cattle gain weight on grain; they make more milk and cream eating roughage, that is, grass and hay. For beef farmers, then, grass means a slower return—cattle fatten much faster on grain—but the farmer also has lower feed costs, more nutritious beef, and a higher price in the right markets. For dairy farmers, grass farming is remarkably efficient. Cream from grass-fed cows contains more omega-3 fats and vitamin A, and spring and fall grass yields significantly more cream. In one survey, Vermont graziers earned more per cow than even the most profitable confinement dairies.

The environment benefits from grazing, too. Industrial grain and soybeans for cattle feed are grown with fertilizer and pesticides, but grass and hay are easily grown without chemicals. Well-grazed pastures have more diverse plants than fallow land. The constant cutting and regrowth of grazing stimulates dense root growth, improving soil fertility and preventing erosion, and because cows walk around, manure is spread evenly, reducing nitrogen runoff.

Livestock and poultry that feed on grass are healthier for several reasons. Fresh air and ample room prevent infection and disease. Instead of standing in their own manure, pastured animals move away from it, preventing the spread of manure-borne diseases. Poultry that follow sheep and cattle eat fly larvae in manure before they hatch, reducing fly-borne illness. Pasture contains many nutrients for animal health, including beta-carotene, selenium, and vitamin E.

In one study, 58 percent of feedlot cattle and only 2 percent of pastured cattle had campylobacter.[11] The *Journal of Dairy Science* reported that 30 to 80 percent of conventional cattle carry *E. coli* in their stomachs, but when cattle were switched from a high-corn diet to hay, *E. coli* declined a thousandfold in only five days.[12] In other words, a mere five days of feeding grass and hay to beef cattle before slaughter will restore the stomach to its normal acidity and kill *E. coli*, which would prevent many cases of contamination in the slaughterhouse. Unfortunately, this sensible, inexpensive practice has not been widely adopted by feedlots.

GRAIN-FED BEEF AND *E. COLI*

E. coli is much feared and misunderstood. Large numbers of the bacteria dwell in the colons of healthy cows and humans, where they are quite harmless. Contamination in the slaughterhouse (usually from fecal matter) is how *E. coli* finds its way into food. If we do eat *E. coli*, our stomach acid usually kills it. But a new, dangerous form, *E. coli O157*, has evolved in the unnaturally acidic gut of grain-fed cattle. Highly resistant to acid, it can survive in our stomachs, so it's more likely to make us sick. *E. coli O157* is *not* found in grass-fed cattle.

Farmers, animals, and the environment all benefit from grass farming. What's in it for steak lovers? Grass-fed beef contains less fat, more CLA, and more omega-3 fats than grain-fed beef. Like game, grass-fed meat has the right ratio of the omega-3 to omega-6 fats (about 1:1), while grain-fed meat is too rich in omega-6 fats. Traditional beef contains more vitamin A and E and more of the antioxidants lutein, zeaxanthin, and beta-carotene. It contains alpha-lipoic acid, an antioxidant essential for cell metabolism, which also lowers blood sugar and improves sensitivity to insulin. Other foods from pastured animals, including bison, lamb, pork, poultry, eggs, and milk, also contain more omega-3 fats, vitamins, and antioxidants than their industrial counterparts. (For more information, see www.eatwild.com.)

Let's take a closer look at the polyunsaturated omega-6 fat CLA mentioned in chapter 2. Though there is some CLA in pork and poultry, this fat is all but unique to the fat—not the muscle—of ruminants raised on grass; that means beef fat and butter. I've touted grass-fed beef and milk for being rich in omega-3 fats and said that grain-fed beef has too many omega-6 fats. CLA is an exceptional omega-6 fat, in that it tends to act like an omega-3 fat. CLA reduces triglyceride and atherosclerosis.[13] It also aids weight loss, reduces body fat, and increases lean muscle, apparently by its effects on lipase, the enzyme used to digest fat.[14]

Other omega-6 fats (mostly in polyunsaturated vegetable oils such as corn oil) *promote* tumors, but CLA, an antioxidant two hundred times more powerful than beta-carotene, *prevents* cancer.[15] CLA slows the growth of tumors of the skin, breast, prostate, and colon.[16] In 1991, *Cancer Research* reported that CLA is "more powerful than any other fatty acid in modulating tumor development."[17] In 2003, researchers who found a link between *cured* meat and cancer noted that grass-fed beef and butter were "almost the only sources" of CLA, the only natural fatty acid the National Academy of Sciences regards as showing "consistent" antitumor effects.[18] *Nutrition and Cancer* reported that "a diet composed of CLA-rich foods, particularly cheese, may protect against breast cancer."[19]

THE GREAT AMERICAN BURGER IS GOOD FOR YOU

Made with grass-fed beef and raw milk cheddar, served on a whole wheat bun with ketchup and a traditional fermented dill pickle.

Beef

Alpha-lipoic acid, essential for metabolism; lowers blood sugar and improves insulin sensitivity

CLA, an omega-6 fat that fights cancer and builds lean muscle tissue

Omega-3 fats, which prevent obesity, diabetes, and heart disease

Stearic acid, a saturated fat that lowers LDL

Vitamins E and A

Bun

Fiber, folic acid, and B vitamins

Ketchup

Lycopene, an anticancer agent

Cheese

Omega-3 fats and vitamin A

Enzymes and beneficial bacteria

Pickle

Vitamins B and C and enzymes

Grass farming is nothing new, of course. Some thirty thousand years ago—before we settled down to farm—we were proto-shepherds, corralling and herding flocks for meat and milk. The patron saint of modern grass farmers is André Voisin, a French dairy farmer and biochemist who wrote the classic work *Grass Productivity* in 1957. The sequel, *Soil, Grass and Cancer*, is a compelling treatise on grass and health. His chapter titles are all poetry, yet each one is also a scientific gem. "The Soil Makes the Animal and the Man" sums up his philosophy of soil fertility, animal health, and good food, while "The Estrogens of Grass" explains why spring grass boosts milk yields.

In a lament called "No Attention Is Paid to the Origin of Milk Used in Experiments," Voisin reminds us that many studies are useless without knowing, say, how putting cows on quality clover affects the nutritional quality of the milk. His own research showed that good Gruyère, a hard cheese made high in the Swiss Alps since 1100, depends on milk from grass-fed cows. Leave it to the Cartesian French to define precisely what makes a great cheese.

The Virtues of Beef, Pork, and Poultry Fat

LET CHEFS AND FOOD CRITICS gush over the sensual pleasures of butter and cream; they are much more eloquent than I am. This chapter is devoted to their unsung health benefits.

All natural fats—polyunsaturated, monounsaturated, saturated—perform important roles in the body. The popular fable, in which saturated fats are the villain, is mistaken. We'll look at these taboo fats again later, but for now, these are the headlines: saturated fats fight infections, aid digestion, and extend the use of the critically important omega-3 fats. Without saturated fats, the body cannot absorb calcium or build cell walls.

You wouldn't learn any of this from reading government advice about what to eat. Lean meat and unsaturated oils are king and queen of the official dietary kingdom. In 2005, the U.S.

government revised its dietary guidelines, and among the key recommendations were these: "Most meat and poultry choices should be lean or low-fat" and "most of the fats you eat should be polyunsaturated or monounsaturated."

Fat is *verboten*. Indeed the word *fat* itself seldom appears in official advice, except in the terms *low fat* and *nonfat*. The section on fats and oils on the USDA dietary guideline Web site is now simply titled "Oils." The USDA's selective exclusions of "fat" are not only misleading; they are a willful rewriting of dietary history. Of the "common" oils listed—canola, corn, cottonseed, olive, safflower, soybean, sunflower—all but one (olive) is a modern oil with a brief history in the diet. These oils have been "common" for perhaps one hundred years—if that long—while we've eaten animal fat for three million years.

"After several decades of vilifying fat and cholesterol, it is now realized that life is not so simple," writes Nichola Fletcher in "Hunting for Fat, Searching for Lean," an essay for the 2002 Oxford Food Symposium, a prestigious gathering of food thinkers. From the Stone Age until recently, fat was the measure of good eating. Fletcher quotes a wistful seventeenth-century peasant: "If I were a king I would drink nothing but fat."

By the middle of the twentieth century, all that had changed, and fats were considered dangerous. Then something curious happened. Just as we began to cast a suspicious eye on fat, we made farm animals—particularly beef cattle—*fatter* by feeding them grain. Moreover, by depriving cattle of the grass that gave their meat omega-3 fats and CLA, we changed the *kind* of fat attached to our steak. The result was beef with more fat, and more saturated fat—the very things medical wisdom now considered killers.

The experts are right: fats are important to health. But we've pointed the finger at innocent fats and overlooked the culprits.

The industrial diet contains fewer omega-3 fats, less CLA, more refined vegetable oils, and (infinitely) more trans fats than our ancestors ever ate—a perfect recipe for diabetes and heart disease. Fletcher concludes that the traditional fats in fish, wild game, and grass-fed beef and dairy are best: "Old fat fine," she says simply. "New fat nasty."

In a moment we'll take a brief tour of the fats found in beef, pork, and poultry. Before we do, it's helpful to understand two things. First, all fats are a blend of three fatty acids: polyunsaturated, monounsaturated, and saturated. But for convenience we describe the fats by the *predominant* fatty acid. Thus we call beef fat saturated, even though it also contains a good amount of polyunsaturated and monounsaturated fats. Second, the more saturated the fat, the firmer it tends to be, and the better for cooking. Chemically, saturated fats are more stable when heated than monounsaturated fats, and polyunsaturated oils are the least stable, and thus easily damaged. This is important, because damaged fats are unhealthy. With those things in mind, here's a fresh look at the benefits of the old-fashioned farmhouse fats.

Not long ago, fast-food restaurants made french fries in beef fat, because it's mostly saturated and monounsaturated and thus stable when heated. For health, beef fat was better than the polyunsaturated vegetable oils they use now, which are easily damaged by heat, becoming rancid and carcinogenic, especially when used repeatedly. A few food lovers remember the superior, savory flavor of french fries made with beef fat.

Beef fat is typically 50 to 55 percent saturated and about 40 percent monounsaturated oleic acid, the same fatty acid found in olive oil, which lowers LDL while leaving HDL level. Much of the saturated fat is stearic acid, which also lowers LDL. As we've seen, the fat of grass-fed beef is a rare source of the anticancer omega-6 fat CLA, which also builds lean muscle. Beef from cattle raised on grass also contains significantly more polyunsaturated omega-3 fats than industrial grain-fed beef.

We once regarded lard as an economical health food. Americans remember eating lard sandwiches with fried onions on homemade bread during the Depression. In lean times, Asians ate a soup of lard (rich in vitamin D) and soy sauce (made of fermented soybeans rich in B vitamins). Like all hardship dishes, it's *almost* nutritionally complete.

Lard is about 50 percent monounsaturated, 40 percent saturated, and 10 percent polyunsaturated, which makes it mostly (60 percent) *un*saturated. As with beef, the amounts vary with the diet of the pig, which is not a fussy eater. In the tropics, for example, where pigs eat coconut, pork is a source of lauric acid, a powerfully antimicrobial saturated fat all but unique to coconut oil. Lard contains about 44 percent monounsaturated oleic acid and 12 percent saturated stearic acid, which lowers LDL.

One of the traditional American cooking fats, lard has a neutral flavor to suit any dish, sweet or savory. (Those who don't eat pork tend to cook with beef and poultry fat.) Lard makes superb, flaky pie crust and biscuits. Because it's mostly unsaturated, lard is relatively soft at room temperature, and it melts and mixes more easily than the more saturated beef fat. To make it firmer and to extend its shelf life, most commercial lard is hydrogenated, the same process used to make solid margarine from liquid vegetable oils. Like all hydrogenated fats, hydrogenated lard contains unhealthy trans fats.

HOMEMADE LARD IS EASY

Making lard is quick and easy, and it keeps for months in the refrigerator. First, find a farmer or butcher who sells "leaf lard" (the abdominal fat that surrounds the kidneys), which has superior, finer texture for baking. Cut the lard in pieces and run it through a food processor. In a heavy pan, melt it over low heat or bake at 325 degrees Fahrenheit until the fat has melted, about twenty minutes. Strain the fat into a glass jar and chill rapidly to keep it clear. The crispy bits are delicious; Italians call them ciccioli and eat them with bread or polenta. If you don't fancy making your own, ask farmers and butchers for unhydrogenated lard. Niman Ranch and some shops sell lardo, a Tuscan specialty of cured fat from the thickest part of the fatback. Use it for sautéing and to flavor sauces.

Poultry fat is as diverse as poultry and the foods they eat. Mostly monounsaturated—and thus fairly heat-stable—poultry fat is also suitable for cooking. Duck and goose fat are traditional in Jewish kitchens and justly honored by French cooks, especially for roasted potatoes. Chicken fat—*schmaltz*, the Yiddish word for fat—is a staple in Jewish recipes, including chopped liver and crispy *gribenes* (chicken skin fried in chicken fat). I once met a man who grew up eating homemade *gribenes* at the movies. (Think of them as kosher pork rinds.)

Poultry fats also contain a few saturated and polyunsaturated fats; again, the diet of the bird affects the composition of the fat. Pastured chickens and poultry fed fish oil or flaxseed oil have more polyunsaturated omega-3 fats, while tropical chickens, like pigs, eat saturated fats in coconut oil. Typically, chicken fat is about 40 percent monounsaturated oleic acid, which lowers LDL. Goose fat is mostly monounsaturated, too (56 percent), as is duck fat (46 percent). Turkey fat contains 38 percent oleic acid, 22 percent polyunsaturated fats, and 22 percent saturated palmitic acid, which lowers total cholesterol and LDL.[20]

We have seen that saturated fats fight infections. All poultry fats, particularly chicken fat, also contain palmitoleic acid, an antimicrobial *mono*unsaturated fat. That's why chicken soup—not skinless chicken breasts—is known as the Jewish penicillin: those pale yellow droplets in chicken broth boost your immunity.

So the next time someone eating a poached skinless chicken breast tells you that your choice of beef, bacon, or roast chicken with the skin will send you to an early grave, this is your reply. First, explain that beef contains stearic acid, which lowers LDL, and that pork and poultry fat are mostly *mono*unsaturated, just like olive oil. Second, say that *natural* saturated fats—as opposed to *industrial* saturated fats, or trans fats—are good for you anyway. In the heat of a dinner party debate, you will probably remember only one good thing about saturated fats. Make it this one: they are powerful immune boosters. Once upon a time, I used only olive oil. When I added butter and other saturated fats to my diet, I stopped getting sick. And yes, the chefs and food critics are right: my cooking was much tastier, too.

I Try the Winston Churchill Diet

Hannah Bantry,
In the pantry,
Gnawing at a mutton bone;
How she gnawed it,
How she clawed it,
When she found herself alone.

—Mother Goose

A MAN OF APPETITES, with the constitution of an ox, Winston Churchill lived to ninety smoking cigars, drinking champagne, and relishing bone marrow. The English have long considered unctuous bone marrow on toast a delicacy as well as a tonic for the malnourished. In London today, the signature dish at St. John—the celebrated restaurant near Smithfield, the wholesale meat market that clatters with butcher hooks in the small hours—is Roast Bone Marrow and Parsley Salad. Chef Fergus Henderson, dedicated to elemental, frugal, and traditional English food, made "nose to tail" eating fashionable.

Marrow may be the oldest and simplest dish ever. Stone Age hunters devoured it even before they went for the raw meat. In Latvia, successful hunters still celebrate by eating the raw bone marrow on bread with salt, pepper, and onion before they divvy up the kill. Organ meats—also called offal or variety meats—have a similar poor-relation reputation, coming in second to more glamorous cuts of pure muscle, such as a T-bone. Yet this distinction between classy steak and down-market liver and bones—not to mention beyond-the-pale parts, like brain and thymus glands—is recent. Dishes built on bones and variety meats fill old American and European cookbooks, and our taste for these foods goes back long before that.

"Since prehistoric times, man and other primates have killed for the valuable fats present in brain, tongue, and marrow," writes the food historian Nichola Fletcher.[21] "Red meat, although prized, was once secondary." Native Americans sometimes returned from buffalo hunts with nothing but tongue. Loren Cordain, the expert on Stone Age nutrition, writes, "There is absolutely no doubt that hunter-gatherers favored the fattiest part of the animals they hunted and killed."

One reason our ancestors preferred organ meats and bone marrow is the sheer desire for fat. Fat is tasty for a host of reasons: because fat kept us alive during long winters, because without fat a woman cannot get pregnant, because fats are essential for digestion. But the particular fats in the oddball cuts are perhaps even more important. They are not, as many people believe, mostly saturated. "Brain is extremely high in polyunsaturated fats including . . . omega-3 fatty acids," writes Cordain. "The dominant fats in tongue and marrow are the cholesterol-lowering monounsaturated fats."

Eating bone marrow had a profound effect: it separated us from our ape cousins and helped make us uniquely human. The human brain grew very large relatively quickly on a diet of long-chain polyunsaturated fats found in bone marrow (and fish, as I describe in chapter 4). Polyunsaturated fats, so vital to brain and visual development, are considered the main factor in our astonishing leap ahead, brain-wise, over other primates. They were still eating mostly fruit, leaves, and insects, while early humans went for fat.

It's too bad that bone marrow is underappreciated. I like to roast beef or lamb shanks and scatter the hot meat on a watercress salad before tossing the bones in the stock pot. Tearing thin shreds of meat off the bone like Hannah Bantry is the fun part; it feels so primitive. Perhaps you don't fancy the role of the clawing, gnawing Hannah—who, let's admit, is cast as slightly uncivilized. Another way to get at the nutrients in marrow is by making broth from bones. A staple of most cuisines, stock adds flavor to starches, richness to soups, and depth to sauces. Fresh stock, which lasts several days in the fridge and freezes well, is also convenient; a bowl of hot consommé with bread makes a quick meal. "Stock is everything in cooking," said Escoffier. "Without it, nothing can be done."

It's also affordable. If you would like to eat well on not very much money, buy soup bones. Broth made from the lesser cuts—necks, knuckles, wings, feet—is rich in minerals including calcium, magnesium, and phosphorus, all in a form that's easily absorbed. Joints are particularly rich in gelatin, called a "protein sparer" because it helps the body use the smaller amounts of incomplete and low-quality protein found in plants. That's why stock is a staple of protein-poor cuisines. Wartime ads for Bovril bouillon cubes in Britain featured a cow made of vegetables because a bit of Bovril (essentially, reduced beef stock) could stretch even vegetables into the nutritional near-equivalent of meat. Stock is also famously good for convalescents. A South American proverb says, "Good broth will resurrect the dead."

I Am Skeptical That Red Meat Causes Cancer

CANCER IS ON THE RISE, and, like heart disease, it has many causes. Damage to DNA increases with age, for example, so our long lives may be one reason for higher cancer rates. Is our diet killing us? My guess probably won't surprise you: I doubt that foods we've eaten for millions of years cause cancer. Indeed, cancer is rare in groups where wild meat is eaten liberally. I tend to suspect industrial foods and chemicals.

The suggestion that animal foods cause cancer took root in 1965, when Dr. Ernst Wynder of the American Health Foundation said that animal fat and colon cancer were linked in the United States and elsewhere. "Unfortunately," said the lipids expert Mary Enig, the consumption data Wynder cited for the United States were "mostly processed vegetable fat," not animal fat.[22] If Enig is right, Wynder's conclusions were unfounded. Enig says that other data undermining the link between animal fat and cancer were neglected or ignored over the years. In 1973, for example, National Institutes of Health researchers looked at diet and cancer in Japanese Hawaiians. "They actually found that the highest risk relationship came from macaroni, green peas, green beans, and soy," writes Enig. Yet the authors concluded colon cancer was linked to beef.

Because cancer is on the rise and red meat is a regular part of diets in most of the industrial world, many researchers have examined a possible link between eating red meat and cancer. Lately, it looks rather weak. In the 1990s, three studies with rats found no relationship between red meat and cancer, but two called for more study on fat itself, as opposed to lean meat. The first study concluded that lean beef did not cause colon cancer.[23] In the second, researchers who fed cancerous rats lard, olive oil, beef, chicken with the skin, or bacon found that beef did not promote tumors.[24] A third group reported that their data "do not support the belief that red meat consumption increases the risk for colon carcinogenesis."[25] They, too, fed rats with cancer various fats (corn oil versus beef fat) and various proteins (lean beef versus milk protein). Rats who ate beef had significantly fewer colon tumors.

Recent human studies don't seem to support the link either. In the 1998 *Australian Journal of Nutrition and Dietetics*, researchers reviewed many published studies, asking "Does Red Meat Cause Cancer?" They concluded that "any true effect of meat is likely to be small, or even an artifact of a decreased consumption of fruit, vegetables, and cereals among high meat consumers."[26] Other researchers reviewed five studies including eighty-three hundred deaths among seventy-six thousand people. The subjects included a large number of vegetarians. There were no differences between the vegetarians and omnivores in death rates from stomach, colon, lung, breast, or prostate cancer.[27] In 2003, a team led by Dr. Walter Willett, the prestigious epidemiologist at the Harvard School of Public Health, followed more than eighty-eight thousand women for eighteen years and found no evidence that eating meat was associated with breast cancer.[28]

Other studies, however, *have* shown a link between meat and cancer. Some researchers suspect that cured meat, not meat itself, is responsible. One of the world's largest studies on diet and health is the European Prospective Investigation into Cancer and Nutrition (EPIC). For cancers of the colon, rectum, stomach, and upper digestive tract, EPIC found fish was beneficial, red meat harmless, and preserved meat harmful.[29] Two studies in Argentina, where people eat a lot of red meat, linked cured meat and colon cancer. Others reported that preserved meats (cold cuts) were linked to cancer, while lean meat was beneficial.[30] Yet another study found that total meat intake was unrelated to colon cancer and large amounts of cold cuts increased the risk.[31]

If cured meat is to blame, the actual culprit may be nitrite, which improves the flavor of cured meat, preserves its pink color, and prevents bacterial growth. Nitrite in various forms has been used to preserve meat since the Middle Ages. Scientists say that nitrites are harmless at the levels we eat them, but at high temperatures nitrites are converted to nitrosamines, which may cause cancer. Nitrosamines are "powerful DNA-damaging chemicals," writes Harold McGee in *On Food and Cooking*. "Yet at present there's no clear evidence that the nitrites in cured meats increase the risk of developing cancer." The use of nitrite has fallen drastically since the 1970s, and fairly small amounts are used now.

McGee is a scientific man, an accomplished cook—and a moderate on meat. "To the extent that meat displaces . . . vegetables and fruits that help fight heart disease and cancer, it increases our vulnerability to both," he says. In addition to nitrosamines, two other carcinogens are formed when meat is cooked at high temperatures.[32] McGee suggests that we eat vegetables liberally and and cook meat gently.

To that good advice, I would add: never burn the fat (if it's smoking, it's burning) and cook meat rare. Even better—if you have a taste for it—make steak tartare and eat it raw. After all, our ancestors ate everything, even fish and red meat, uncooked for about three million years before they first used fire, only 250,000 to 350,000 years ago. For raw meat dishes, Sally Fallon recommends using frozen beef as a precaution against parasites. For steak tartare, I only use grass-fed beef from a farm I trust. I also buy nitrite-free bacon and salami.

If not meat, what dietary factors might account for the rise in cancer? For me, the simplest approach is to ask what's *new* in the diet, and fats are key. Industrial food contain too many omega-6 fats and too few omega-3 fats, an imbalance that promotes cancer, according to omega-3 experts, including Dr. Andrew Stoll and Dr. Artemis Simopoulos.[33] Wild game, grass-fed meat, and grass-fed butter—until recently, the only kind—contain omega-3 fats and CLA, the powerful anticancer fat.

Another major factor in cancer is lack of antioxidants, including vitamins C and E and the hundreds of compounds in fruits and vegetables. The interactions of foods are mightily complex. Here's a curious one, again from McGee: fruit, vegetables, and acidophilus bacteria in yogurt appear to diminish the effect of the carcinogenic compounds formed when meat is burned. Anyone—vegetarian or omnivore—who eats a lot of fruits and vegetables is doing the right thing.

One other hypothesis about cancer and fat deserves more study—especially because some research exonerates *lean* meat. Modern life is rife with carcinogens, from plastics to pesticides. Stone Age humans certainly had their worries, but persistent environmental toxins weren't among them. Some believe that cancer comes not from animal fat itself but from the "bioaccumulation" of carcinogens in the fat. As toxins travel up the food chain, they become more concentrated, and they lodge in fat. A feedlot steer contains a great deal of grain, most of it grown with chemicals, which means you ingest more chemicals from a steak than from a slice of bread. Any toxins in the beef fat, in turn, accumulate in *your* fat, which might explain the rise in fat-related cancers. As ever, the sensible thing is to avoid foods laden with chemicals.

Buying and Cooking Real Meat

ONCE YOU GET THE hang of it, buying and cooking grass-fed and pastured meat and poultry is easy. Here are the essential facts about the labels *grass-fed*, *pastured*, and *organic*, and some kitchen tips.

Grass-fed applies to ruminants: cattle, sheep, goats, and game. It means animals were raised on grass and hay, but how much varies widely; the term is not legally defined. Ideally, fresh pasture makes up the bulk of the diet, and when there's no grass, animals eat hay. Some farmers add a dollop of sorghum silage, which many would regard as a grass-based diet, or corn silage. However, silage is fermented—sort of like sauerkraut for cows—and fermented foods, like grain, give cattle an acid stomach. Purists never feed silage, grain, corn, or soybeans to ruminants.

Grain-finished beef was raised on grass and fattened with grain. I can live with a little silage or grain in my beef—even a wild steer would have eaten a few seed heads—but if you're a purist, look for the label *100 percent grass-fed*.

Pastured applies to pork, poultry, and eggs when animals are raised on pasture. "Grass-fed" bacon and eggs is not correct, because a diet of grass isn't enough for these omnivores. Like humans, pigs and chicken need complete protein. Pastured chickens eat corn, insects, and sour milk as well as grass. On eggs or poultry, the label *vegetarian feed* is misleading. It means chickens were not fed other ground-up chickens—and that's good. But chickens are not natural vegetarians. What it *does* mean is the birds never went outside; if they had, they might have eaten a grub or two. *Free-range* poultry and eggs says nothing about grass. It means the birds aren't in cages, but they may be in barns or on bare dirt. Grass is the key source of beta-carotene, CLA, and omega-3 fats in pastured poultry and eggs.

As I've mentioned, there is no single diet for the not-picky, omnivorous pig. Swine will eat different foods on every farm: acorns and apples here, coconut and corn there. Whey-fed pork is popular on dairies because farmers have plenty of protein-rich whey to spare after cheese making. Pigs are sometimes raised in barns on deep straw; this is better than industrial pork, but ideally pigs root outside in meadows or woodland, usually with huts for shelter. Good fencing is the key; it is not easy to keep pigs from running riot. If a local farmer raises pastured pork, count yourself lucky and eat up.

LETTING PIGS GO HOG WILD

Beverley Eggleston of EcoFriendly Foods in Moneta, Virginia, explains how pigs like to live: "Wild hogs are foragers with a great sense of smell; they root with strong snouts. Pig and plow come from the same root word. You will never find a happier pig than one up to his shoulders in dirt, chewing on wild potatoes or other roots. I've seen pigs flip big rocks over with their noses, just for fun. Our farmers raise hogs in a setting that allows them to run around and dig. Because pigs literally tear up the landscape, it's important to use that to the advantage of the farm, not the destruction. The industry's solution is to put the pigs on concrete; this makes a boring and hard life for the pig. On the other hand, you can't really put them on pasture and expect the grass to last. The obvious solution is to put the pigs in a place that you want to dig up anyway."

Organic is legally defined. It means the food was produced without synthetic fertilizer, antibiotics, hormones, pesticides, genetically engineered ingredients, and irradiation. Organic does *not* mean animals were grass-fed or pastured. Organic beef, pork, and poultry eat organic grain, but most commercial versions are not raised on grass, or their access to pasture is minimal.

Conversely, *grass-fed* and *pastured* don't mean animals were raised to organic standards, but the grass farmer who uses antibiotics, hormones, pesticides, or genetically engineered foods is rare. The label *natural* says nothing about the animal's diet. It means the product contains no artificial flavor or color, chemical preservative, or any other artificial ingredient. This weasley term is widely used. According to the USDA, "all fresh meat" qualifies as "natural."

In the 1950s, when corn-fed beef became trendy, good cooks adjusted their recipes—or so I imagine. Similarly, you may need to tweak things a bit for lean grass-fed beef. Many people believe that lean meat is bound to be tough, but the grass-farming expert Jo Robinson says that fat marbling accounts for only 10 percent of variation in tenderness. Other factors are breed, cut, age, and sex of the animal, calcium levels in the soil (and thus the meat) whether it was stressed before slaughter, how it was chilled (too cold and it toughens), how long it was hung, and, of course, how you cook it.

"We would no sooner cook salad bar beef like fat beef than we would cook venison like fish," says Mr. Grass himself, Joel Salatin. The chief risk with grass-fed beef and bison is overcooking. At high temperatures, the proteins in meat contract and toughen. Grass-fed steaks cook in half the time of a grain-fed steak. Other things being equal, the lower the final temperature of the meat, the more tender it will be.

That said, there are two approaches: cook it very quickly and keep it rare; or cook it slowly, with moisture. For steak, the food writer Betty Fussell, an expert on beef, favors quick cooking over high heat. "Rare should be really rare," she says. "If you like a buttery texture, add a pat of herbed butter to the cooked steak, French-style." Some cooks marinate steak first. With other cuts, cook it low and slow, with moisture. As with any meat, the less tender cuts, such as chuck steak, benefit from braising.

You may need to make other minor adjustments with grass-fed meat. When you calculate how many people a roast will feed, you don't need to allow for shrinkage—grass-fed tenderloin, for example, is so lean that very little fat is lost—but the temperature should be lower and the cooking time shorter. When browning grass-fed ground beef for chili or spaghetti sauce, I find it helpful to use a fair bit of olive oil.

Industrial beef is fattier than traditional beef, but with pork, the opposite is true. Commercial pork has been bred very lean—that's why kitchen tricks to prevent dry meat are often called for—and traditional pork is richer. The industrial pig is typically 56 percent lean, while Bill Niman, founder of Niman Ranch, favors 48 to 51 percent lean pork. A fatter and moderately muscled pig has more flavor.

Many small farmers raise a standard commercial breed like the Large White. A Yorkshire native, the Large White has been a registered breed in England since 1884, and it has proved adaptable on modern farms. It does well in confinement and produces a great deal of bacon and other cuts from its straight back and large loin. Other farmers favor rare traditional breeds like Gloucester Old Spot, Large Blacks, and Tamworths, which are often richer than conventional breeds. A loin of pastured Gloucester Old Spot requires very little doctoring. A little olive oil, salt, rosemary, and a very hot oven will do nicely.

Pastured chicken has a rich flavor and firm texture compared with flabby and insipid factory chicken. Stock made from pastured chicken is superior, too. I suspect that's because a chicken that gets exercise on well-managed pasture and grows slowly has more gelatin in its joints, more amino acids (protein) in its meat, and more minerals in its bones. In other words, a pastured chicken is a more complex and dense creature, and that makes for richer, tastier, and more nutritious stock.

Recently, poultry breeds have won more attention from farmers and chefs. The typical commercial chicken is a large-breasted Cornish cross, and many small farmers raise it on pasture. Other farmers raise traditional, slow-growing breeds such as Redbro, Mastergris, or GrisBarre, which tend to be leaner, with darker meat and rich flavor. Traditional turkey breeds, once endangered, are also making a comeback. Look for Standard Bronze, Narragansett, Royal Palm, Bourbon Red, and Black Slate.

Cooking pastured poultry is simple: just watch the leaner breeds to avoid dry meat. They benefit from shorter roasting times and the sort of tricks used on wild fowl, such as wrapping with bacon. I'm a fan of traditional turkey breeds, but for roast chicken, I find some of the older breeds a bit too skinny, so I tend to buy a commercial breed, like a Cornish cross. When raised on pasture, they seem to have the right combination of meat, juice, flavor, and tenderness.

4

Real Fish

How Our Brains Grew Fat on Fish

WHAT WOULD YOU SAY to a six-year-old who asked you: where do farmers come from? Perhaps you would tell a bedtime story like this: Back in the Stone Age, our ancestors were skillful hunter-gatherers. They gnawed on marrow bones, dug tubers, gathered seeds, cracked nuts, and speared fish. Life was good. Over time, however, the smarter ones perceived that a little planning and organization would yield a more reliable food supply, one that could be more easily stored for a rainy day and shared with others. These innovative deer hunters and berry pickers began to tame smaller wild cows and plant larger seeds of wild grass. Eventually, the tribes who were best at these new tricks put aside their restless ways and settled down in villages to harvest grain and herd animals for milk and meat. They became farmers.

Richard Manning has a subtly different take on what he calls the "just so" story of the rise of agriculture. He believes fishing was the second-oldest profession, not farming. In *Against the Grain*, Manning imagines early humans were keen to be near a steady supply of eels, salmon, and other migrating fish. They looked for neighborhoods with good water and rested there to wait for hordes of fat seasonal fish; only *then* did they start to tend, guide, herd, and harvest wildlife in the backyard. While waiting for the river mouth to disgorge fish, the Cro-Magnon had time to paint the mighty salmon on cave walls, a sure sign of its importance.

Fishing man—call him *Homo piscator*—fills in part of the story of the transition from swinging in the trees (like our fruit-loving primate cousins) to becoming hunter-gatherers and, eventually, farmers. Paleoanthropologists have long puzzled over the "missing link"—the ancestor we share with chimpanzees and gorillas, whose bones (mysteriously) are not found in the fossil record. Where did they live, how did they move about, what did they eat? No one knows.

In 1960, the marine biologist Alister Hardy offered a novel theory about the era after we came down from the trees and before we settled on the plains. Suppose we spent a few million years living in the shallow waters of the sea, like aquatic mammals including the dolphin, hippo, and sea cow? According to Elaine Morgan in *The Descent of Woman*, the quasi-aquatic ape hypothesis could explain a number of downright peculiar human features: nude skin, subcutaneous fat, always plump breasts, how newborns love to swim, why we have sex face-to-face . . . I could go on about the ways we are unusual among primates. But for our purposes, the most compelling thing about the idea that our ancestors once lived in the water is our dramatic and indisputable dependence on fish.

If you've glanced at a biology text recently, you'll know that the river ape idea is not widely accepted. However, the experts do agree our taste for fish is ancient. Many fossils tell us that some two million years ago, at least three hominid species lived near the huge freshwater lakes of the East African Rift Valley. Each had its niche. The ones with broad, flat molars apparently ate a plant-based, high-fiber diet; another group, with smaller teeth, ate mostly small fruit, berries, and the occasional egg or rodent. The third species, of course, was our very own *Homo habilis*. Dubbed "handy man" for the tools he used, including fishing gear like spears and nets, he was an omnivore—and loved fish.

Whether we lived in it or near it, water offered easy access to DHA and EPA, omega-3 fats essential to visual, mental, metabolic, and hormonal function found only in fish. The body can make its own DHA and EPA from another omega-3 fat found in plants, Alpha-linolenic acid (ALA), but the conversion of ALA to DHA and EPA is inefficient. Making DHA and EPA requires vitamin B_6, magnesium, calcium, and zinc; it is hindered by trans fats, cortisol, alcohol, and sugar.[1] Moreover, the plant sources of ALA—walnut, flaxseed, and canola oil, and a weed called purslane—were not abundant in the Stone Age. Then, as now, the best source of these vital fats is fish. This is a dilemma for vegetarians; in the future, DHA and EPA supplements made from algae may solve it.

DHA and EPA are vital to the brain. Like bone marrow, which helped our brains grow much bigger and faster than the brains of leaf eaters, fish was brain food. Recall that the brain is 60 percent fat; *half* the fat is DHA.[2] Dr. Andrew Stoll puts it bluntly in *The Omega-3 Connection*, "Without large amounts of DHA . . . we might not have evolved at all." No wonder the search for fish and seafood is universal. The overwhelming bulk of the human family has settled near sea shores and river mouths. The exceptions—landlocked and mountain people—go to great lengths to trade with fishing groups for seafood.[3] Like the bonobo—our closest relative, a playful creature that likes to catch shrimp with its hands—*Homo sapiens* is a water-loving ape.

Life After Salmon: Obesity, Diabetes, and Heart Disease

THE KLAMATH RIVER RUNS through the mountains of northwest California, passing through the town of Happy Camp, home of the Karuk tribe. Once the Klamath River ran thick with salmon, which the Karuks devoured at every meal, each one putting away more than one pound of fish daily. Then, in the 1960s and '70s, hydroelectric dams stopped the water, the salmon disappeared, and the Karuks turned to industrial foods.[4]

When wild salmon were plentiful, diabetes and heart disease were rare. Not now. The percentage of tribe members with diabetes has risen from near zero to 12 percent, almost twice the national average. Forty percent of the tribe has heart disease—three times the national rate. "You name them, I got them all," Harold Tripp, a Karuk fisherman, told the *Washington Post*. "I got heart problems. I got the diabetes. I got high cholesterol. I need to lose weight."

That's what happens when people lose access, almost overnight, to traditional foods and must resort to poor-quality foods. In this case, the nutritional mechanisms are well understood. Omega-3 fats prevent the trio of modern diseases—obesity, diabetes, and heart disease—in multiple ways.

Let's look first at the effects on metabolism, because metabolic disturbances are in many ways the root of all three conditions. Omega-3 fats regulate blood sugar levels and fat burning. DHA and EPA in particular are directly involved in activating the expression of genes controlling fat metabolism. For example, mice fed the same number of calories from fish oil are leaner than those fed corn oil, which is rich in omega-6 fats. People whose muscles are low in omega-3 fats are more likely to be obese.

Obesity, in turn, leads to diabetes. In the United States today, diabetes and metabolic syndrome—or prediabetes—are epidemic. "In medical school, I was taught that if you can understand diabetes, you will understand all of medicine," says Dr. Andrew Stoll, author of *The Omega-3 Connection*, "because those with diabetes fall prey to many other disorders, from cardiac disease to kidney failure to stroke."

What is diabetes? When blood sugar rises, the pancreas secretes the hormone insulin, which signals the muscles to take sugar from the blood to muscles. Once in the muscle, the sugar has two uses: as immediate energy or as short-term, stored energy, in the form of glycogen, which marathon runners draw on. In type 1 diabetes, the pancreas does not produce insulin at all. In type 2 diabetes, which accounts for 90 to 95 percent of cases, the pancreas does produce insulin, but the muscles don't respond; they are "insulin resistant." When the muscles are deaf to insulin, sugar, which is toxic at high levels, gathers in the blood. Until recently, type 2 diabetes was viewed as an adult disease, and it is still most common in overweight people over fifty-five, but the rising number of cases in children is a distressing trend. Diabetes, it seems, is not a disease of age, but of diet. Fish is important, because omega-3 fats decrease insulin resistance.

EAT FISH TO BEAT INFLAMMATION

In type 1 diabetes, the body attacks its own pancreatic cells. Other autoimmune diseases include arthritis, psoriasis, Crohn's, lupus, colitis, and asthma. A common symptom is chronic excessive inflammation. Omega-3 fats prevent inflammation, and omega-6 fats promote it. Dr. Artemis Simopoulos (*The Omega Diet*) says the protective effect of omega-3 fats on autoimmune kidney disease is "one of the most dramatic effects of omega-3 fats on any pathology."[5]

Diabetes, in turn, leads to heart disease. According to the cardiologist Dr. Arthur Agatston, author of *The South Beach Diet*, half of heart disease patients have metabolic syndrome first. The evidence that omega-3 fats prevent heart disease is robust and growing. Omega-3 fats reduce the risk of a first heart attack and reduce the risk of sudden death during a heart attack by 20 to

40 percent.[6] The Physician's Health Study, which followed twenty thousand doctors, found those eating fish as little as once a week were half as likely to have a fatal heart attack as those who ate fish less than once a month.[7]

If you've survived one heart attack, eating fish can prevent another. The *Lancet* reported a study of more than two thousand men who had recovered from a heart attack and were given various instructions on diet. Advice to reduce fat made no difference in mortality, but men told to eat fatty fish two or three times a week had 29 percent fewer deaths from all causes—the most important measure in epidemiology. Researchers called the effect "significant," even after adjusting for ten potentially confounding factors.[8]

Such studies always cheer me up. All too often, nutritional research is ambiguous, the results are modest, and the advice is . . . well, *confounding*. Happily, the news on fish is good and getting better. If you're lucky enough—as the Karuks once were—to live near a source of wild salmon, take advantage of it. Not so lucky? See "Where to Find Real Food," on page 276.

HOW OMEGA-3 FATS PREVENT HEART DISEASE

- Raise HDL
- Reduce LDL and VLDL (very low density lipoprotein)[9]
- Reduce blood pressure by dilating the blood vessels
- Reduce clotting, inflammation, and triglycerides
- Reduce lipoprotein (a),(Lp(a)) which promotes atherosclerosis and blood clots[10]
- Reduce risk of death during and after heart attack by reducing irregular heartbeat (arrhythmia) through the actions of sodium, calcium, and potassium ions in heart muscle

Are You Depressed? Try Eating More Fish

MUSCLE AND BONE ARE made of protein and minerals, but the brain is the house that fat built. Our brain is particularly hungry for the omega-3 fats found in fish. While other organs can manage (if not ideally) on a ratio of four parts omega-6 to one part omega-3 fats, the brain appears to require equal amounts of each.[11] Why? Unlike other body tissues, the brain can't make DHA and EPA from plant oils like walnuts and flaxseed. In nutrition jargon, the brain has an "absolute need"—as opposed to a conditional one—for DHA and EPA, which, as we've seen, are found only in fish. Without adequate DHA and EPA, brain cell membranes don't function properly. Abundant research, much of it recent, confirms that fish is food for thinking. In 2005, for example, the *Archives of Neurology* reported that older men and women who eat more fish have sharper minds and better memory.

Mental health is one of the most exciting therapeutic applications of fish oil. Omega-3 fats may be as powerful as the drugs a psychiatrist prescribes, even for serious depression. Population studies, lab work, and clinical experience with depressed patients all suggest that fish oil can prevent and treat depression. The omega-3 expert Dr. Joseph Hibbeln has found that differences in depression rates across countries can be predicted by the quantity of fish in the diet. Lab analysis shows that the brains of depressed people have less omega-3 and more omega-6 fats. Finally, clinical evidence is mounting: doctors have prescribed omega-3 fats for major depression, postnatal depression, bipolar disorder, and schizophrenia, with impressive results.

The risk to mental health of omega-3 deficiency starts in the womb and continues throughout life. The baby has massive needs for DHA and EPA, especially in the second half of pregnancy, when growth is mostly due to fat.[12] Formula-fed babies and those nursed by omega-3-deficient mothers fail to develop proper visual and mental function. Premature babies are particularly vulnerable because they are poor converters of ALA to DHA and EPA. In one study, premature babies fed corn oil had underdeveloped eyes and poor vision, while premature babies fed fish oil were virtually identical to full-term, breast-fed infants. Thus, even when the situation is not ideal—preterm infants are at greater risk in many ways—fish oil can make a difference.

QUALITY OF BREAST MILK IN SAMPLE POPULATIONS

In addition to mental and visual problems in the baby, lack of omega-3 fats causes preeclampsia, eclampsia, premature birth, low birth weight, difficult labor, and postnatal depression. Note how much the quality of breast milk varies, presumably with fish consumption.

Breast milk	*Ratio of omega-6 to omega-3*
Ideal milk	1 to 1
Inuit, Canada	3.8 to 1
Coastal China	7.1 to 1
Japan	9.9 to 1
Urban China	24.4 to 1
Rural China	28.2 to 1
United States*	67.4 to 1
United States*	175.0 to 1

*Two studies were conducted in the United States.

Source: Andrew Stoll, *The Omega-3 Connection.*

In children, omega-3 fat deficiency is linked to dyslexia, poor motor skills, and attention deficit hyperactivity disorder.[13] Deficient teenagers and adults are prone to anger, hostility, and violence. Pregnant and nursing women who don't replenish omega-3 stores face serious risk of postnatal depression.[14] (Omega-3 fat depletion is cumulative; that is, if the mother's diet lacks these essential fats, deficiency grows with each pregnancy and each generation.) In older people, lack of omega-3 fats is linked to Alzheimer's disease and dementia.

Fish oil prevents depression in several ways. Omega-3 fats make up nerve cell membranes, which affect the transmission of nervous system signals. ALA, DHA, and EPA regulate calcium, sodium, and potassium ions, which control electrical activity in the brain. Omega-3 fats directly activate receptors for neurotransmitters including dopamine and serotonin, chemical messengers for mood, sleep, appetite, and libido—symptoms altered or crippled by depression. Finally, eicosanoids have a vital (though poorly understood) effect on mood.

Schizophrenia is one of the more distressing and intractable mental illnesses. The traditional treatment, which is more than fifty years old, employs drugs to alter levels of dopamine and serotonin. This works for about 30 percent of patients—not impressive. Moreover, the drugs are costly and cause side effects. A radical new approach begins with the observation—first suggested by Dr. David Horrobin in the 1970s—that the brain is made of fat.[15] Neurotransmitters are carried in pouches made of fats called phospholipids, which the body can make from plant-based sources of omega-3 fats or (ideally) obtain directly from fish. In the schizophrenic brain, however, the complex metabolism of fatty acids is damaged, so that neurons and neurotransmitters don't work properly. Early clinical trials suggest that fish oil supplements might be as effective as drugs, without the side effects.[16]

If fish oil can prevent or treat obesity, diabetes, heart disease, and depression, the muscular salmon immortalized by Cro-Magnon artists begins to look like a delicacy, superfood, and wonder drug, all wrapped up in one speckled silver package.

Clearly, eating fish is a good thing. If only deciding *which* fish to eat were as simple.

The Truth About Fish Farming

FISHING IS FUN, but—famously—it involves a fair bit of waiting around for the fish to fall into the trap, whether it's a net, basket, or hook. If you fish for fun, simply watching the water rush by is pleasant enough, but it would quickly seem inefficient if dinner depended on it. One day, a clever *Homo piscator* (his brain swollen by omega-3 fats) began to wonder whether there wasn't a quicker, more reliable way to gather the tasty protein he was now accustomed to eating every day. His idea was to trap, feed, and breed fish. In Asia, carp farming is an ancient form of agriculture; the book *Fish Culture Classics* was printed in 460 BC.

Alas, traditional fish farming is all but forgotten. The marine equivalent of cattle feedlots, confinement dairies, and battery egg farms, fish feedlots present the all-too-familiar problems of intensive food production: crowding, disease, parasites, pesticides, antibiotics, excess manure, environmental damage, and—did you guess?—less nutritious food. Just as beef, milk, and eggs raised on grass contain more omega-3 fats than those fed grain and soybeans, wild fish contains more omega-3 fats than farmed fish.

These undesirable effects were little known in the 1970s, when the Norwegians pioneered salmon farming. Quickly taken up by Scotland, Chile, and Canada (all countries blessed with long, indented coastlines), fish farming was an immediate hit. "By the late 1980s, salmon had gone from being a luxury fish to an absolute steal," writes Gina Mallet in *Last Chance to Eat*. No doubt that seemed like progress, but the effects on salmon, the sea ecology, and nutrition were less savory.

WILD FISH BETTER THAN FEEDLOT FISH

	Wild		*Farmed*	
	Grams of fat	*% of omega-3*	*Grams of fat*	*% of omega-3*
Salmon	10	20	16	17
Eel	21	14	30	12
Trout	5	30	6	20

Source: Artemis P. Simopoulos, "Omega-3 Fatty Acids in Health and Disease and in Growth and Development." *American Journal of Clinical Nutrition*, Vol 54 (1991): pp. 438–63.

The insults start at birth. To stock fish feedlots, female and male salmon are anesthetized before farmers squeeze out their eggs and sperm. Like the animals on factory farms, farmed salmon is fattier than wild fish—by design. The feedlot diet of fish meal and growth-promoting antibiotics is deliberately fattening. Wild fish also get a lot more exercise, which produces firm, well-toned flesh, not the flabby, greasier version found in feedlot fish.

Wild salmon is measurably cleaner than feedlot fish. In 2004, *Science* published research showing that farmed salmon contains "significantly" more toxins, including PCBs and dioxin, than wild fish. Similar problems occur in other farmed seafoods. Imported farmed shrimp may contain the drug chloramphenicol. This potent antibiotic drug is used in therapeutic doses for treating serious infections in humans. The United States does not permit chloramphenicol to be used on animals or in animal feed.

Thanks to its natural diet of shrimp, wild salmon is a rich pink color. The species called sockeye is the richest in the carotenoid astaxanthin, a powerful antioxidant. Feedlot salmon, however, is naturally gray. To give farmed salmon the hue we crave, fish farmers rely on a dye called canntaxanthin. "The color is chosen from Salmofan," says Mallet, "a color swatch from the chemical giant Hoffman-La Roche."

It was first thought that aquaculture would protect wild fish, but it turned out to be the other way around. Today more than half the world's salmon is farmed, and the majestic species known as Atlantic salmon is hanging by a thread. In the icy waters of Alaska, on the other hand, where salmon farming is banned, the result is a world-famous, thriving wild salmon fishery. Crowded industrial fish are more susceptible to parasitic sea lice, which (despite routine pesticides) easily spread to wild fish. Each year, millions of salmon escape from feedlots and breed with wild fish, reducing genetic diversity.

Fish farming also causes collateral ecological damage. Feedlots produce chemical runoff from antibiotics, pesticides, and detergents, and tons of fish feces, too much to be cleared by ocean currents. In Asia, Latin America, and Africa, shrimp farming is destroying the complex and vital ecosystem found in mangrove swamps.

The industry defends fish farming as a source of cheap, high-quality protein. However, like other industrial crops, fish feedlots represent a net *loss* of energy. About three pounds of wild fish are consumed to produce one pound of farmed salmon or shrimp. In *Against the Grain*, Richard Manning describes the unfortunate logic of the industrial fish food chain.

> The protein that supports this practice comes from what we call "trash" fish, such as sardines and herring . . . Many of these species, however, are not trash at all, but a key link in the ocean's food chain and an important part of local fisheries and diets in the developing world. Left to their own devices, wild fish (especially salmon) eat the fish that factory trawlers are now scooping up and grinding into fish meal to feed to farmed fish. Absent the trawlers, local fishers in skiffs . . . would catch a few anchovies to

feed local protein-starved communities. Instead, this protein is sucked up, reduced by a factor of three, and shipped to Red Lobsters across suburban America.

The fish we *should* farm are herbivores (carp, catfish, tilapia) and mollusks (oysters, mussels). But there is money in the carnivores (cod, salmon, shrimp, tuna). Happily, there are a few environmentally sound alternatives to industrial fish farms. Scotland and Ireland raise organic salmon without antibiotics and pesticides; they use lower stocking densities, organic feed, and a natural pink dye, typically made from ground-up shrimp. Scotland also offers sustainable farmed cod, and shrimp from Ecuador are certified organic by Naturland.

ECO-FRIENDLY FISH AND SEAFOOD

Conservation organizations, including the Blue Ocean Institute and the Audubon Society, rate fish and seafood by its abundance and the ecological impact of fishing methods. Find current editions of this guide from the Monterey Bay Aquarium at www.seafoodwatch.org.

Best choice	*Not bad*	*Avoid*
Catfish (farmed)	Clams (wild)	Caviar (wild)
Caviar (farmed)	Cod: Pacific	Chilean seabass
Clams (farmed)	Crab: blue	Cod: Atlantic
Crab: Dungeness	Crab: king (Alaska)	Crab: king (imported)
Halibut: Pacific	Flounder: summer/fluke	Grouper
Lobster: spiny (U.S.)	Lobster: Maine	Halibut: Atlantic
Mussels (farmed)	Mahi Mahi	Monkfish
Oysters (farmed)	Oysters (wild)	Orange roughy
Salmon (wild)	Pollock	Red snapper
Sardines		Salmon (farmed)
Shrimp (trapped)		

Striped bass
Sturgeon (farmed)
Tilapia (farmed)
Trout: rainbow (farmed)
Tuna (troll/pole-caught)

Scallops: bay and sea
Shrimp (U.S. farmed)
Sole (Pacific)
Squid
Swordfish (U.S.)
Tuna (long-line caught)

Shark
Shrimp (farmed or trawler)
Sole (Atlantic)
Sturgeon (wild)
Swordfish (imported)
Tuna: bluefin

Most American wild salmon comes from the Pacific. The premier species is sockeye, whose rich ruby color signals high levels of the natural antioxidant astaxanthin, but some people prefer the milder and richer king salmon. From the Lower Fraser River in Washington State comes the marble chinook, the only really regionally distinct species, which is caught by hook and line or trolling, often by Makah and Nootka tribes. The best-quality fish is frozen on the boat, ideally before rigor mortis—when enzymes begin to break down the flesh—sets in. Fish "frozen at sea" is regarded by people in the know as superior to never-frozen fish—unless, of course, you live near water and your fish goes straight from the sea to the skillet.

Here in New York City, I often buy local seafood, but I also cook wild Alaskan salmon from small independent boats, a choice I regard as socially and environmentally sound. It is certainly preferable to any farmed salmon. My red sockeye come from the *Tommyknocker*, the boat of Rosemary McGuire, who fishes Alaska's famous Copper River Flats. Filets and steaks arrive frozen in vacuum packs and taste of the sea. The hot smoked salmon in jars is exquisite. I also love wild Alaskan sablefish. Sometimes called black cod or butterfish, you often see it smoked, in Jewish delis. Ivory and flaky, sablefish has a buttery texture, delightful flavor, and 50 percent more omega-3 fats than salmon. Filets frozen at sea are superb, but for every day, I eat a lot of canned wild salmon, which is not expensive.

It's sensible to eat fatty fish two or three times a week—and when you do, be generous with the butter and cream. Saturated fats extend the body's supply of omega-3 fats; hence classics like Dover sole with butter sauce, lobster claws dipped in melted butter, and creamy clam chowder. Cold-water, oily fish (mackerel, herring, bluefish, salmon, tuna) have the most omega-3 fats. A 3.5-ounce (100 gram) portion of sockeye salmon contains more than 1,200 milligrams of DHA and EPA. Sardines—a catch-all term for any young fish, often herring—contain 500 percent more omega-3 fats than tuna.

A word of caution about wild fish, however. Mercury is an environmental pollutant known to cause brain damage. Like other metals, mercury accumulates in tissue as it moves up the food chain, which means larger, carnivorous fish contain more mercury than smaller ones. Thus the FDA advises children and pregnant women not to eat swordfish, shark, king mackerel, or tilefish. But it's unwise to avoid fish altogether.

Why? The benefits of fish to mother and baby are "enormous," says Dr. Michel Odent, an expert in prenatal nutrition.[17] Odent is concerned that more women fear excess mercury than understand how important fish oil is. In 2005, a study by the Harvard School of Public Health confirmed this view, arguing that the mercury warnings could cause pregnant women to eat too little fish, not only for the baby's brain but also for their own health. "I think we've got two messages," said Joshua T. Cohen, who led the research. "If you're not pregnant and you're not going to become pregnant, eat fish. If you are pregnant or you are going to become pregnant, you should still eat fish, but you should eat fish low in mercury.'[18]

Like the FDA, Odent advises pregnant women to avoid the big carnivorous fish, and encourages women to eat plenty of the small, fatty ones, like the anchovy, pilchard, herring, and common mackerel. Mostly herbivorous, farmed fish such as catfish, carp, trout, and tilapia are also good choices if mercury is a concern. The jury is out on tuna, a carnivore; the cautious pregnant woman might prefer to avoid it. If you don't care for fish, do take a high-quality fish oil, in capsules or liquid.

WHERE FISH KEEP OMEGA-3 FATS

Oily fish (salmon, tuna, mackerel) store omega-3 fats in muscle. The soft brown flesh beneath salmon skin is a particularly rich source. Flaky white fish store omega-3 fats in the liver. I can buy monkfish liver, a Japanese delicacy, at my local farmers' market. Sauté it in butter and put a slice on toast. The French call it *le foie gras de la mer*. The best supplement is the traditional favorite of old-school nannies: cod-liver oil, rich in omega-3 fats and vitamins A and D. Some brands have a mild citrus flavor. Another good choice is wild sockeye oil. All fish oil should be wild and unrefined. Quality fish oil supplements don't contain mercury or PCBs.[19]

Should you eat fish raw? Yes—traditional diets include a lot of raw fish. The Inuit eat mostly raw seafood and blubber, the Japanese love sashimi, the Spanish make seviche, and Scandinavians have gravlax (salmon cured with sugar, salt, and dill). These recipes make nutritional sense because polyunsaturated omega-3 fats are very sensitive to heat. According to Stoll, when you cook a piece of fish, the omega-3 fats are partially protected by lower temperatures in the middle. Nevertheless, the less heat

5

Real Fruit and Vegetables

Why I Never Rebelled Against Vegetables

FARMING IS RELENTLESS; my father calls it a "vegetable-driven existence." Our season started in March, with tomato seedlings in the greenhouse. In April, we picked the always-thrilling first crop (I still love spinach for that reason), and soon after came the more glamorous strawberries and rhubarb. When the June heat hit, zucchini production exploded, cucumbers were next, and blueberries came in on the Fourth of July. In the height of summer, we picked and sold hundreds of bushels of tomatoes.

After Labor Day, we had to pick sweet corn before school, and when we came up the hill from the bus stop in the afternoon, a note on the kitchen table told us where to pick beans. By late September, we were all half praying for an early, hard frost to end our vegetable-driven days, but the cool-weather crops were still to come. In October, we lugged baskets of butternut squash, and our hands got numb from washing turnips and collard greens in big tin buckets. For vegetable farmers, winter is a great relief, like silence after listening to jack hammers. I don't know how dairy farmers keep going twelve months a year.

You might expect a childhood like that to put me off vegetables forever. But I love everything about them: how pretty they look on the plant, picking them when they're just right, even washing, chopping, and cooking them. Most of all, I love to eat vegetables; I know there are a few I don't like, but without effort I can't remember what they are. Salsify, maybe—but then I never seem to cook it properly. And white asparagus.

At the farm in high summer, abundance is the norm. The fields, the cool basement, and the kitchen are filled with the finest varieties of the freshest vegetables you'll ever taste, and maybe that's why I eat more vegetables than anyone I know. For a salad to serve two, I use a large head of lettuce. Whatever we're having for dinner—pork loin, sautéed chicken livers, fish—I usually make at least two vegetables, often three or four. On my own, I often make an entire meal of vegetables, usually with some richer topping, like butter, walnuts, or blue cheese.

There's no nutritional advice more dog-eared than "Eat your vegetables," but that won't stop me from repeating it here. A heap of solid evidence shows that a diet rich in fruits and vegetables helps prevent macular degeneration, age-related decline, heart disease, and cancer. Fruits and vegetables are packed with good things, including fiber, potassium, and vitamin C, but the exciting research is on huge classes of antioxidants like carotenoids and flavonoids. Scientists have identified four thousand different flavonoids alone; the task of learning what each one does, and how, is gargantuan.

The research tidbits emerging about phytochemicals (plant chemicals) are fun for the produce-obsessed. For example, anthocyanins, the flavonoids in blackberries and blueberries, are the most powerful antioxidants of 150 flavonoids.[1] Tart cherries are another nutritional gold mine, with seventeen different antioxidants, including two powerful anthocyanins not found in blueberries or cranberries. In Michigan, they swear by Montmorency cherry juice to beat pain and inflammation from arthritis and gout. It's also delicious.

A RAINBOW OF GOOD THINGS

Carotenoids—fat-soluble compounds that protect plants from the sun and our cell walls from attack by free radicals—are the most famous antioxidants in plants, but there are thousands of others. Here, some potent antioxidants are grouped by color, the catchy organizing principle of books like *Eat Your Colors* and *What Color Is Your Diet?* By the way, I don't use the microwave, which destroys antioxidants, enzymes, and vitamins dramatically more than conventional heat.

Yellow and green

Spinach, peas, and avocados

Lutein and zeaxanthin help prevent cataracts and macular degeneration

Orange

Carrots, mangos and sweet potatoes

Alpha-, beta-, gamma-, and zeta-carotene fight cancer, and beta-carotene prevents LDL oxidation

Red and pink

Tomatoes, pink grapefruit, and watermelon

Lycopene lowers LDL and helps prevent lung disease and prostate cancer

Red and purple

Blueberries, grapes, red cabbage, and red peppers

Anthocyanins delay cellular aging and reduce blood clots

Have you noticed that most natural poisons, from hemlock to deadly nightshade to toadstools, are found in plants, not in meat, fish, and eggs? Plants are rooted to the ground and can't run from predators, so they need other defenses. Plants respond to an invasion (or prevent one) by making bitter compounds called phenolics. Insects like aphids dislike the taste of phenolics, so they abandon the plant for other food. Scientists have identified some ten thousand compounds designed to foil the hungry animals who would devour plants, including alkaloids (potatoes), tannins (tea), and oxalates (rhubarb).

"Plants produce these weapons only if they need them," writes the naturalist Susan Allport in *The Primal Feast*. Watercress, for example, is peppery yet sweet when young but turns bitter when it flowers, just when it needs to keep insects at bay to make seeds for the next year. The same is true of lettuce. Once hot weather hits, lettuce bolts; instead of sending tender leaves *out*, it shoots a firm stem straight *up* to prepare a seed head. As any gardener knows, once the lettuce has bolted—I love the term, which suggests fleeing the scene on short notice—it turns bitter.

Some of the bitter compounds in plants, such as strychnine (part of the alkaloid family) are toxic to humans. In large quantities, the green blush on potatoes left out in the light is poisonous, as are rhubarb leaves. But many phytochemicals are powerful antioxidants and very healthy. Bitter herbs, often represented by horseradish, have a prominent place on the Passover plate. I like to ponder the material reasons for enduring culinary traditions, and this one certainly makes nutritional sense. All leafy greens are good for you, bitter ones especially so.

GOOD FAMILY NAMES

When you know the value of whole plant families, it's easier to shop for the foods you prefer. If you don't fancy a stir-fry of beef and broccoli, get your phytochemicals from leek soup, roasted turnips, or watercress salad with blue cheese.

The Alliums

Actually members of the lily family, onions, garlic, leeks, and scallions contain allicin, an antibiotic that fights tumors, reduces cholesterol, prevents blood clots, and reduces blood pressure.

The Aster Family

The asters include lettuce, endive, radicchio, chicory, and dandelions. This would be easier to remember if you ever saw a lettuce flower; it looks like a little dandelion or wild aster. They're digestive tonics and rich in beta-carotene.

THE CHICORIES

- Belgian endive (missile-shaped with cream-colored, yellow-tipped leaves)
- Radicchio (typically round, with rich pink, densely packed, curvy leaves)
- Puntarelle (wild chicory spears, dressed with oil, lemon juice, garlic, and anchovies in Italy)
- Dandelion (quite bitter and worth adding to salads)

THE ENDIVES

- Curly endive (frilly, green and yellow head; also called frisée)
- Escarole (a broad-leafed endive that looks like romaine)

The Genus *Brassica*

Also called the mustards, Brassicas include broccoli, brussels sprouts, cabbage, cauliflower, collards, horseradish, kale, kohlrabi, mustard, turnips, and watercress. They contain beta-carotene and sinigrin, which fights colon cancer.

THE NASTURTIUMS

- Watercress (*Nasturtium nasturtium-aquaticum*) and the flowering garden nasturtium are Brassicas but deserve a special mention because they're too little appreciated. Watercress and nasturtium (leaves and flowers) are peppery and lovely in salads. Rich in beta-carotene and vitamin C, watercress is a mild stimulant, diuretic, and digestive tonic.

Curiously, we are the rare animal that actually likes the bitter taste of radicchio or black tea. I fear, however, that Americans raised on sugary soft drinks are losing the taste for things savory, sour, and bitter. It's pitiful that commercial salad dressings contain sugar, and even sweet corn hybrids are much sweeter than when I was little. We're not alone. In Britain, plant scientists are breeding sweeter hybrids of the brussels sprout, famous for its dour presence at Christmas lunch, but the more palatable sprouts may lack the healthy, bitter compounds.

In the kitchen, the classic complements to "bitter herbs" such as turnip greens, frisée, and Belgian endive are rich ingredients with equally strong flavors: salty fatback and pancetta, pungent Roquefort. These toppings make nutritional sense, because the body needs fat to convert the antioxidant beta-carotene into usable vitamin A. When you make a mess of greens (as they say in the South), don't stint on the fatback; they belong together.

Thinking about our funny, plant-driven childhood, I asked my brother, Charles, what he remembered about meals on the farm, and right away he mentioned one of my most vivid associations: red raspberries and Sunday mornings. At six AM we picked raspberries for the Takoma Park farmers' market, which starts relatively late, at ten AM. (For selling delicate produce, nothing beats a sign saying PICKED TODAY.) After the market truck left, we picked another pint or two for raspberry-studded pancakes. The syrup was simply berries boiled with sugar until they fell apart.

We grew other small fruit, too: black raspberries, blueberries, tart cherries, and strawberries. I love them all. Now we grow only one strawberry—a little thing with a short season called Earliglow—because we've never found a better one. We feel about Earliglows as William Butler, the sixteenth-century English physician, felt about strawberries. "Doubtless God could have made a better berry," he said, "but doubtless God never did."

Berry picking is a pleasant job, even when you are picking for market, and I am a fast berry picker. I also have a sharp eye for spotting wild fruit. On the farm, I know the fencerows where furry wineberry bushes lurk and where to find mulberry trees drooping with white or purple blobs. Finding berries in baking-hot suburban parking lots or running along old canals is fun, too. In New York, my local mulberry tree is only blocks away, in a little park on the East River.

Plants, as we've seen, make themselves bitter out of self-defense. Berries, likewise, dress up pretty out of self-interest. The vivid crimson and blue of wild raspberries, blueberries, and cranberries must have popped out like jewels to the hunter-gatherer eye. From the plant's point of view, looking lovely draws the attention of animals, who will then eat the fruit, travel, and spread the seeds—a neat trick if you're a blackberry bush and can't walk around. For the forager, meanwhile, sapphire and ruby clusters are like the bitter taste of dandelions: they signify good things, including vitamin C and anthocyanins.

When I see quarts of dark sweet cherries at the farmers' market or glimpse a purple splotch in a tangled green fencerow, I smile and cheer up a little. I like to think that's my Stone Age brain, perking up.

What Is an Industrial Tomato?

WHEN WE PICTURE INDUSTRIAL MEAT, the images are unpleasant: animals crammed on concrete floors in dark barns, tails docked, getting fat on hormones—and that's about right. It's more difficult to conjure up an industrial tomato. Sure, large commercial farms probably don't look like a backyard garden, but how badly can they mistreat a simple tomato? In fact, the traditional and industrial tomato have little in common.

Before the first seed is sown, soil is sterilized with fumigants like methyl bromide, which is toxic to wildlife and people. Healthy soil is never sterile; it should be teeming with fauna, from earthworms and nematodes to microbes. Soil fertility—and thus plant health—depends on the interaction of these organisms with the soil and plant roots. A teaspoon of grassland topsoil may contain twenty million fungi and five billion bacteria, creatures who want to be fed with minerals, compost, and other organic matter. On industrial farms, however, soil life is not nurtured; it's murdered.

The seeds are different, too. Industrial varieties have traits convenient to large growers, distributors, and retailers. An industrial tomato, for example, is bred to be solid and thick-skinned, the better to tolerate mechanical harvesting, washing, packaging, and long-distance shipping. Uniform shape and size are also important. Flavor and texture take a backseat. Gardeners and small farmers prefer great flavor to good looks, not that the two qualities are mutually exclusive.

Industrial farming also favors monocropping, but single crops, as the Irish learned the hard way with potato blight in 1845, are more susceptible to devastation by pest invasion and disease. The industrial answer is herbicides, fungicides, and pesticides to kill weeds, insects, and molds. So powerful are these chemicals, industrial farmers have dispensed with crop rotation—the age-old method for keeping pests and disease at bay—but the apparent efficiency is illusory. With this system, pests and pathogens traditionally kept in check by switching crops accumulate, thus requiring yet more pesticides.

As with factory animals, rapid, high yields are the goal on industrial produce farms. Synthetic fertilizers, especially nitrogen, make plants grow fast, but nitrogen-driven growth produces weak, watery, and overly leafy plants which are more vulnerable to insects. Furthermore, most of the nitrogen runs off, polluting streams, rivers, oceans, fisheries, and drinking water.[2]

Industrial farmers use hormonelike chemicals to push plants to grow bigger and set fruit faster. Almonds, broccoli, grapes, melons, onions, potatoes, snap beans, tomatoes, and other crops may be treated with growth enhancers such as AuxiGro. Rather like a steroid for plants, it promises enhanced flowering, larger fruit size, and greater yields—with what effect on texture, flavor, and nutrition, I don't know. We do know that steroids enhance performance in cattle and baseball players, and we know the extra beef, milk, and muscle come at a price. Plants have equally delicate hormonal systems.

Harvest is different on industrial and traditional farms, too. Industrial peaches and plums taste nothing like local ones in season, in large measure because they're underripe. Industrial fruits cannot be picked ripe; they would never survive the journey, often thousands of miles, to the supermarket. Industrial tomatoes are picked "hard green" and ripened artificially with ethylene gas. They never develop the complex flavor or luscious texture of a tomato that ripens naturally, with just the right combination of acids and sugars, like a balanced wine.

Another difference between industrial and ecological produce is postharvest treatment and packaging. Most treatments are designed to make produce look fresh longer. But is it still fresh? En route to shops, produce is irradiated to kill bacteria such as *E. coli* and extend its shelf life. Irradiated strawberries can still *look* fresh after three weeks, long after an untreated berry would have spoiled. That certainly helps the supermarket produce manager, but irradiation destroys vitamins, and with every day it sits on the shelf, the berry is less tasty and nutritious. According to Public Citizen, irradiation also produces new compounds called alkylcyclobutanones, which are linked to cancer and genetic damage in rat and human cells. Groceries, meanwhile, promote irradiation as a public health measure. But I don't want sterilized food; I want food that's clean in the first place—and still alive.

How "baby" salad leaves got trendy is one of my favorite industrial produce stories. First, supermarkets offered washed leaves as a convenience to cooks. (By the way, the history of laborsaving devices in the American kitchen is not encouraging, and I doubt that people who are too busy to wash lettuce enjoy more leisure than I do.) But the prewashed cut leaves turned brown too quickly, so growers started to sell small, whole leaves, which lasted longer because they weren't cut.

This convenience to industrial lettuce growers, produce wholesalers, and supermarkets was presented as a gourmet delight—baby spinach!—but to me, it's simply immature and tasteless. Nor am I a fan of "micro" greens—and they seem to be getting younger all the time. I saw "infant" arugula on a fancy menu recently, but I prefer mine all grown up.

Adding injury to insult, cut salad leaves are often packed in Modified Atmosphere Packaging (MAP). After the leaves are washed in chlorine, they're put in bags with less oxygen and extra carbon dioxide. The result is lettuce that still looks fresh ten days to a month later.[3] Unfortunately, MAP lettuce contains fewer vitamins C and E and antioxidants. Any cut lettuce loses nutrients quickly, but, as with irradiated berries, MAP lettuce still looks fresh after ten days, while untreated lettuce has withered and turned brown—a sure sign that it's past its peak and thus unsellable.

Let's return, briefly, to the unpleasant topic of pesticides. Of all the unsavory aspects of industrial produce, pesticides, though invisible, are probably the most dangerous. "The fact that spreading billions of pounds of toxic pesticides throughout the environment each year results in extensive harm should not be surprising," writes Monica Moore in *Fatal Harvest: The Tragedy of Industrial Agriculture,* a book of photos of industrial and ecological farms. "Yet somehow it remains not just surprising, but eternally so. This never-ending lack of awareness of the true scale of damage keeps people from challenging assumptions that societies benefit more than they lose from . . . dependence on pesticides."

THE MOST CONTAMINATED PRODUCE—AND THE LEAST

Between 1992 and 2001, the USDA tested forty-six fruits and vegetables for pesticide residue. Using this data, the Environmental Working Group published a list of the least and most contaminated produce. A score of 1 represents the least pesticide residue, 100 the most.

Most contaminated		*Least contaminated*	
Peaches	100	Sweet corn	1
Strawberries	89	Avocado	4
Apples	88	Pineapples	6
Spinach	85	Cauliflower	10
Nectarines	85	Mango	12
Celery	83	Sweet peas	13
Pears	80	Asparagus	16
Cherries	76	Onions	17

Potatoes	67	Broccoli	18
Bell peppers	66	Bananas	19
Raspberries	66	Kiwi	23
Grapes (imported)	64	Papaya	23

Pesticides are bad news. Organophosphates and methyl carbamates, widely used insecticides, can cause acute poisoning, with symptoms including headache, dizziness, fatigue, diarrhea, vomiting, sweating, and stomach pain. Severe poisoning brings convulsions, breathing difficulty, coma, and death. Paraquat, a powerful herbicide, damages the skin, eyes, mouth, nose, and throat; it can destroy lung tissue and cause liver and kidney failure.

Chronic and long-term effects of pesticides include cancer, infertility, and hormone disruption. According to the EPA, 170 pesticides are possible, probable, or known human carcinogens.[4] The common weed killer 2,4-D is linked to non-Hodgkins lymphoma, and lindane (in lice shampoo) is linked to aplastic anemia, lymphoma, and breast cancer. DBCP (a nematode killer) and 2,4-D reduce fertility. The herbicide atrazine is an endocrine disruptor, as is the infamous organochlorine DDT. Though it is now banned in the United States, DDT still lingers in the environment.

We've gone too far. Songbirds are missing, frogs are sterile, and our bodies may already bear the signs of misadventures with powerful poisons. Farmers and their children have higher rates of cancer and birth defects. All these chemicals were designed to kill, after all. One way to reduce your exposure to such nasty things is to eat produce raised with organic or other ecological methods. But what does *organic* mean? And when does it matter?

I Learn How to Answer the Question: *Are You Organic?*

WHEN WE FIRST SOLD at farmers' markets in 1980, they were brand-new to the Washington, D.C., area and pretty new in other American cities, too. New York City's fabled Greenmarket had opened only a few years before, in 1976. People were just getting used to having farmers set up shop in suburbs and cities. It was all new to us farmers, too, of course, but we did our best—even us nine-year-olds. Pictures of me at our motley stand from the early years reveal in embarrassing detail how much we had to learn about display and marketing. We did explain that producer-only farmers' markets (as they're known in our world) were for local farmers to sell homegrown foods, but *local foods* was not yet in the lingo or understood to be a good thing.

The word *organic* was very much in vogue, however. We heard the same question over and over: *are you organic*? We stumbled over various answers, most of them probably beginning like this: "No, but . . ." This reply, as you might imagine, failed to satisfy. First, it sounds defensive. Second, some customers, quite reasonably, were seeking organic produce certified by an independent party, not verbal assurances from a barefoot farm kid.

We felt stuck. We couldn't—and wouldn't—use the word *organic* because we were not certified organic by the state of Virginia, but people wanted to know how we grew our vegetables. One day at the Arlington farmers' market, I was typically flummoxed, when a friendly customer made what must have been an obvious suggestion: that we describe our methods on signs, something like NO PESTICIDES or OUR CHICKENS RUN FREE ON GRASS. Excited, I went home with this idea, which my mother took up with typical editorial intensity, and now our sign boxes are brimming with information.

We had always used ecological methods, such as mulching to

keep weeds down, and we grew most crops without any pesticides, but when we first started farming, we also used some chemicals. We sprayed the weed killer Roundup on pernicious Johnson grass, herbicides on corn, and fungicides on melons (melon leaves prefer dry weather, but Virginia is humid). Soon we gave up all those poisons, but I can still smell the metal cupboard where we kept them. Next time you find yourself in a garden supply store, go to the chemical aisle, and you'll know the dreadful odor I mean.

How much should you worry about the chemicals on produce? Allow me to answer in a leisurely way. When I was little, we ate a lot of industrial produce. In the summer, of course, we ate our own vegetables, but in the winter we bought large bags of industrial fruits and vegetables at Magruder's, the family-owned, local chain famous for good prices. Every day, we ate a large green salad, a fruit salad, or both. My mother insisted.

These days, apart from the occasional mango or avocado, I buy local produce from the farmers' market all year. There are many organic growers, but less than half of my produce is certified organic. I should buy more organic and ecological produce, but for various reasons, I don't. Certain items, like ecological apples and pears, are scarce, and with the huge quantity of produce I eat, price is a factor. Happily, the non-organic growers I know are well shy of industrial. Still, I do miss eating our own vegetables—all well-chosen varieties, grown on mineral-rich soil with strictly ecological methods.

If you can't find or afford ecological produce, *eat plenty of fresh fruits and vegetables anyway*. You may be sure that most studies showing the benefits of diets rich in fruits and vegetables were done on industrial produce. It is sensible to wash industrial produce, but peeling is a tough call. Most of the pesticides are found in, or just under, the peel. So are the vitamins and antioxidants. I simply don't know which is the lesser evil.

When I'm deciding how to spend my food money, I use one other rule of thumb: *the higher up the food chain, the more important ecological methods are.* Thus I spend good money on grass-fed and pastured meat, poultry, dairy, and eggs, but I am less fussy about fruits and vegetables. That's because chemicals accumulate at the top of the food chain, especially in fatty tissue. If there is pesticide residue in, say, a stick of industrial butter, it comes from the many bushels of industrial corn and grain the cow ate.

National organic standards implemented in 2002 made some small organic farmers feel threatened by large-scale organic farming. There is no reason to worry. The new organic rules, if somewhat weak in places, put the spotlight on clean food, and that's valuable. *Organic* means food was produced without synthetic fertilizer, antibiotics, hormones, pesticides, genetically engineered ingredients, and irradiation. In shops, where the consumer is one or more steps removed from the farmer, the organic label is a legal guarantee.

I admire organic farmers, large and small; they're committed to clean methods and willing to subject their farms to independent scrutiny. But many of us—farmers and eaters alike—don't need the organic label. Farmers like my parents, who sell at farmers' markets or to chefs, can explain directly to buyers why the food is superior to industrial produce. Moreover, many farmers use ecological methods that may even exceed the organic standards. For example, they promote healthy plants by adding major nutrients such as calcium, trace elements from sea water, and beneficial microbes to the soil. Cattle farmers raise beef on grass, which yields more nutritious beef than feeding cattle organic grain. But the organic standards don't specify a grass diet. It is up to farmers raising grass-fed beef to tell their story, and that is exactly what they are doing, just as we told our story at farmers' markets twenty-five years ago.

WHEATLAND VEGETABLE FARMS
LOUDOUN COUNTY, VIRGINIA

Our thirty-five acres of vegetables, melons, small fruits, flowers, and herbs are grown without herbicides, insecticides, or fungicides. Since 1980 we have used ground limestone, compost, cover crops, mulches, and a nontoxic, seawater-based foliar fertilizer as our only sources of plant nutrition. Each season we hire college students to help us seed, transplant, mulch, irrigate, pick, load, and sell our crops at twelve producer-only farmers' markets.

—Chip and Susan Planck

We sorely need more research on the nutritional value of industrial and ecological produce. With healthy soil, ecological produce should contain more vitamins, minerals, and antioxidants. At the University of California, Alyson Mitchell compared vitamin C and healthy polyphenols in strawberries, corn, and marionberries (a type of blackberry) grown with organic, sustainable, or conventional methods.[5] The organic and sustainable methods consistently produced higher levels of both nutrients. Unsprayed marionberries and corn had 50 to 58 percent more bitter-tasting polyphenols than conventional produce.

Local food tastes better. Does organic food taste better, too? Sometimes. The important factors of flavor are soil health, variety, maturity, and freshness. Out of necessity, most big organic producers use the same varieties as industrial farmers, pick them underripe, and ship them a long way. It's good that large organic farms don't pollute the rivers, but the tomatoes are tasteless. In Britain, the main commercial strawberry, Elsanta, is known in the trade as the "three-bounce berry." Sturdy Elsanta may be, but it doesn't taste very good, even when it's grown without chemicals. Farmers who care about good food grow varieties with superior flavor, pick them at peak maturity, and sell them fresh. When I hear someone say, "Organic tomatoes taste better," I think, "Which tomato, grown where?"

Farmers have expanded the traditional seasons for local foods with techniques such as row covers, heated greenhouses, unheated hoop houses, and long-season varieties. In New York, I can eat greenhouse salad leaves in snowy January. Tomatoes grown in heated greenhouses—either in a liquid nutritional formula or in soil substitute—appear in the spring, well before field tomatoes, and ever-bearing strawberries are available all summer. For all these foods, we are thankful.

Yet I prefer fruits and vegetables grown outdoors in proper soil in peak season. Soil, which varies from farm to farm, gives produce its flavor and nutrients. That's *terroir*, the French idea that the features of a particular spot—soil type, minerals, moisture, frost—impart special character to the grapes and thus the wine. Environmental stresses—wind, rain, insects—also yield sturdier and more robustly flavored plants. It's a kind of character-building theory of flavor. Hydroponic tomatoes are insipid because they have no *terroir* and no character. If you buy tomatoes out of season, look for those grown in proper soil, often in unheated hoop houses.

Local foods are more diverse than what you find in the supermarket produce section. At my local farmers' market, there are dozens of tomatoes and more than a hundred apple varieties, but supermarkets carry just a few. The eighteenth-century Newtown Pippin, native to the Newtown Creek in what is now Queens, New York, is a superior dessert, cider, and storage apple, but it has been replaced by the rock-hard, often underripe, and less tasty Granny Smith. In October 1785, Thomas Jefferson, who grew 170 varieties of fruits at Monticello, wrote James Madison from Paris, "They have no apples here to compare with our Newtown Pippin."

This lovely apple—now being revived by the equally delightful Ed Yowell, who leads the New York City convivium of Slow Food—has modern fans, too. "The green-skinned, yellow-fleshed Pippin is both sweet and tart; crisp and tender," says Peter Hatch, director of the Monticello gardens. "The citruslike aroma—some describe it as *piney*—lingers in the mouth like a dear memory."

Growing different varieties is also more interesting for the farmer. No one wants to plant, pick, sell, and eat the same zucchini, year after year. My parents grow about a dozen different cucumbers and two dozen varieties of tomatoes, both heirlooms and hybrids. Why grow modern hybrids at all? Aren't heirlooms better? They can be. Let me explain.

The revival of traditional varieties—often from seeds saved over many generations—has been a boon for what the poet Gerard Manley Hopkins called pied beauty. "Glory be to God for dappled things," he wrote. Now we have green escarole speckled with red dots, cucumbers that look like lemons, candy-striped beets, and a tomato that reveals tropical sunsets when sliced. One of my favorites, it's called Pineapple.

Beyond beauty, genetic diversity itself is valuable: a large library of traits gives breeders more material to work with. The Sturmer, an English apple now difficult to find, has five times more vitamin C than Golden Delicious. Americans can thank the Irish potato famine for the Green Mountain potato, an almost-forgotten Vermont native. Around the time of the Irish catastrophe, blight nearly wiped out New England potato farms. Wary of another crop disaster, farmers and breeders developed a blight-resistant variety in the 1880s. For fifty years, the tasty but oddly shaped Green Mountain was America's most popular baking potato, until the more consistently oval Russet took over.

Modern hybrids—which are bred from two parents, thus blending their traits—also have good points, such as high yields, hardiness, and pest resistance. Other qualities I'm less keen on, such as thick skin or excessively firm flesh, are hallmarks of industrial produce. Hybrids per se are not objectionable; after all, breeding is an old and honorable agricultural practice. One laments the loss of useful qualities. When seed companies began to focus on industrial production, flavor and other fine traits were neglected, some lost forever.

Three cheers, then, for seed savers who brought back charmers like Cherokee Purple, a tomato with dark creamy flesh and superlative flavor. We've also grown some lackluster heirloom tomatoes, like Great White and Purple Calabash. Some heirlooms have abysmal yields and poor consistency; even superior flavor may not be enough to make growing them worthwhile. Happily, the renewed demand for flavor and texture has opened the gene libraries of many good seed companies, and that means more and better traditional varieties for farmers to try.

Meanwhile, we're big fans of hybrids like Early Girl, Lady Luck, and Lemon Boy. Dad calls them "garden" hybrids. They taste great and yield well, but for various reasons—small size, delicacy—they don't suit industrial growers, so you won't find them in supermarkets. For me, flavor is tops. I won't spend four dollars a pound on tomatoes merely because they're a wacky color or the sign says HELIRLOOM. They must taste good—and many hybrids do. Yield matters to the cook, too; if I have to cut away large parts of a funny-shaped tomato because of scarring, my salad gets more expensive. With a shapely and reliable hybrid like Lady Luck, that's unlikely.

How to Eat More Vegetables

YOU ALREADY KNOW THAT eating plenty of fruits and vegetables is a good thing. The trick is actually doing it. If you also cook for selective eaters—children or adults—perhaps you worry that they don't eat spinach every day. Relax; no one eats spinach every day. It may help to think not in terms of meals or even days, but rather in weeks. What's important is your overall diet; you won't be malnourished in one day.

Buying local food makes eating vegetables easier and more fun, but if you want to eat more vegetables, it doesn't matter where you shop. Farmers' markets, farm stands, farm shares, green grocers, and supermarkets are all good. These are my tips.

Stock up. If you don't buy produce, you'll never eat it. I tend to be frugal, but in this case, I much prefer to have produce on hand and risk throwing it away than not have any. Buy large amounts of produce when it's cheap, especially during a glut. On most trips to the market, I stock up on basics like lettuce and zucchini, and rarely buy expensive treats such as wild blueberries or fancy mesclun. I find "baby" vegetables overpriced and insipid. At my local market, lettuce is a bargain at one dollar a head all summer; for most of the year, I use two heads a day. There is always fruit in the house for dessert.

Have a salad at every meal. Once you adopt this habit, lunch or dinner without a raw vegetable seems incomplete. If you tire of lettuce, there are lots of leaves: watercress, radicchio, endive, escarole, dandelion, purslane. Try salads of shaved fennel and orange slices or lightly cooked vegetables, as in celeriac remoulade. At the farm, we have a plate of sliced tomatoes at every summer meal. Be aware that some vegetables are more nutritious when cooked. The broccoli and cabbage family contains goitrogens, which depress thyroid function. Spinach, beets, and chard contain oxalic acid, which blocks calcium and iron absorption. Goitrogens and oxalic acid are reduced by cooking. Beta-carotene in vegetables is more available to the body once it has been liberated from tough cell walls; thus shredding, juicing, and cooking beets and carrots are all ways to make them more nutritious.

Dress it up nicely. Say good-bye to plain steamed broccoli. Every vegetable should be properly dressed, and to me that means the right fat, a little salt, and perhaps one flavor, such as fresh herbs or good cheese. When the only fat I used was olive oil, all my vegetables tasted the same. Now I'll make buttered carrots with thyme, roasted zucchini with garlicky olive oil, and a green salad with macadamia oil and macadamia nuts. The vegetables taste better, they taste different, and it's easy to eat all three.

Eat salad first. I happen to prefer the American habit of eating salad before the main course. Raw vegetables stimulate digestion and leave you hungry for the next course. Protein, hot foods, and creamy dishes, by contrast, are satiating. After that sensory experience, you're not hungry for salad anymore. But suit yourself on this one.

Eat salad as a main course. Cobb salad is one of my favorite one-dish meals, but there are many others. Learn to make Caesar salad dressing, buy Romaine lettuce, and do what restaurants do: top it with chicken or shrimp.

Put it out there. We know very little about how eating habits form. Why, for example, do some children develop a diverse palate and not others? You might suspect cultural factors—maybe some parents offer kids cayenne and garlic, others bland foods—but the studies are equivocal. However, it's safe to assume that if you don't put food out, no one will eat it. One small study, hoping to shed light on the eating habits of overweight kids, found that the sole factor predicting how much they ate was the amount of food on the plate. This applies equally to adults. If you want to eat more of something, serve it. My mother set out raw fruits and vegetables before dinner, when we were hungry. In the summer, we had sliced tomatoes and in the winter, a jumble of apple, carrot, and turnip slices.

Eat local food. Here's a paradox. Eating local food leads to *more* variety in your diet, not less. When offered the same global fruits and vegetables all year long, many people get stuck in food ruts. They buy the same fruits and vegetables—bananas and broccoli, or whatever their favorites happen to be—year round. If you buy local food in season, meals will vary without planning or effort. You'll eat spinach in April, strawberries in May, fennel in June, corn in August, and pears in November.

Mix it up. Variety whets the appetite. In fact, science has documented this phenomenon. They call it *sensory-specific satiety.* A fancy term, but all it means is that you're more likely to eat four different vegetables—one creamy, one crunchy, one sharp, one sweet—than four servings of one vegetable. As I write, in the height of July, there are four local fruits in the kitchen: sweet cherries, red gooseberries, blueberries, black raspberries. After lunch, I'll have a bowl of mixed fruit and raw Jersey milk: five foods in one dish.

It's entirely up to you whether you eat more fruits and vegetables. But someone has to be responsible for the nutrition of babies and small children. How much should we worry when they don't eat vegetables? Every parent will have to wrestle with this question, but my best guess is that from zero to two years old, the overriding nutritional requirement is for high-quality fat and protein for growth and development, starting, of course, with breast milk. But the older you get, the more important antioxidant fruits and vegetables are. Why?

Free radicals (unstable atoms with unpaired electrons) are a normal product of cell metabolism, created when cells use oxygen to burn fat. Unfortunately, their numbers rapidly increase with age and damaging environmental factors. Whatever the source, free radicals are highly damaging to cells. They cause the body to oxidize and age, like rusting iron, and contribute to heart disease and cancer. Antioxidants in fresh produce battle the cumulative effects of environmental carcinogens and free radicals.

When your baby starts to eat solid foods, try three simple things. First, steer clear of extra calories from corn oil, juice, and sugar, because any inferior food displaces some more important nutrient. (The easiest way to do this? Don't buy them.) Second, purée the food the whole family is eating, rather than create separate meals for the baby. There is every reason for him to eat a soupy version of homemade spaghetti Bolognese or roasted vegetables; that's exactly what store-bought baby food is. It will be faster than making a separate dish, and cheaper and better than commercial baby food. Third, buy wild fish, ecological produce, and pastured meat, poultry, dairy, and eggs if you can. Children are more vulnerable to pesticides and other toxins than adults.

Otherwise, try to feed children as you would anyone else: with a diverse and balanced diet of whole foods, in hopes of creating good eating habits to last a lifetime. Most kids don't grow up on vegetable farms, and they turn out fine. It would be too bad if children became teenagers still hating vegetables, but it's probably not dangerous. After all, most of us survived our junk-food years.

Suppose you try all of these things and still don't eat enough broccoli and blueberries. Is taking vitamin C and anthocyanin pills good enough? In cases of deficiency, vitamin therapy is safe and effective, and some supplements, like fish oil, are highly beneficial, and consistently so. But there are some questions about vitamin supplements. The results of trials with supplements isolated from whole foods range from unhelpful (smokers taking beta-carotene had higher rates of lung cancer) to promising (vitamin E prevents second heart attacks) to merely equivocal (another vitamin E study on heart disease showed no effect).[6] However, studies consistently find that diets rich in antioxidants from *whole foods* lower risk of heart disease and cancer.

Scientists are just beginning to uncover how extracted vitamins are imperfect substitutes for foods. Whether vitamin E supplements are helpful, for example, has been hotly debated. Why are the studies equivocal? Here's one hypothesis: the vitamin E in supplements is usually alpha-tocopherol, but the vitamin E "complex," as the natural vitamin E in foods like avocados is known, contains at least seven other agents, including beta-, delta-, and gamma-tocopherol. The other agents may be equally or more important. In a similar fashion, the vitamin C in most pills is merely ascorbic acid, but the C complex includes the flavonoid rutin and the enzyme tyrosinase. Without tyrosinase, ascorbic acid doesn't cure fever. Thus, maybe beta-carotene supplements didn't help smokers in that well-publicized study because isolated beta-carotene does not equal a carrot.

Eating fruits and vegetables is still the best preventive measure. They simply don't know how to put all the benefits of foods like beets and broccoli and berries into a pill.

6

Real Fats

Some Surprising Facts About Fats

THE BAD FOR YOU COOKBOOK, published in 1992, in the midst of the frenzy for "light" cooking, extolled lard, eggs, butter, and cream—for pleasure if not health. Chris Maynard and Bill Scheller presented their favorite recipes for shirred eggs, lard pie crust, and trout with bacon with unguarded enthusiasm—and this disclaimer: "As for heart attacks . . . we are not going to make any hard-and-fast recommendations here because we are not doctors and—far more important—we are not lawyers."

How little has changed since then! Many Americans are still terrified of eating fats and feel guilty when they do. Monounsaturated olive oil makes the official list of "good" fats, yet few will defend saturated fats. Traditional fats are certainly more fashionable recently. The television chef and restaurateur Mario Batali made a splash putting *lardo* (cured fatback) on his menus, and food writer Corby Kummer praised lard in the op-ed pages of the *New York Times*. "Here's my prediction," wrote the trend-spotting columnist Simon Doonan in the *New York Observer*, after he saw Kummer's piece on lard. "This trend is not only going to catch on, it's going to sweep the nation."

Well, I hope so. Lard may be in vogue, but hardly anyone knows that lard is good for you. When I began to read about fats with an open mind, I learned some curious things. Consider this: lard and bone marrow are rich in monounsaturated fat, the kind that lowers LDL and leaves HDL alone. Stearic and palmitic acid, both saturated fats, have either a neutral or beneficial effect on cholesterol. Saturated coconut oil fights viruses and raises HDL. Butter is an important source of vitamins A and D and contains saturated butyric acid, which fights cancer. As for the vaunted polyunsaturated vegetable oils, we eat far too many. Refined corn, safflower, and sunflower oil lower HDL and contribute to cancer.

Back when I took the warnings about saturated fats to heart, I cooked everything—from roast chicken to salmon, mashed potatoes to polenta—with olive oil. After I did a little homework on fats, life in the kitchen got more interesting. What fun to rediscover—and in some cases learn for the first time—how to cook with traditional fats like butter and lard. Now my kitchen is stocked with local butter, lard, duck fat, and beef fat, as well as exotic oils of coconut and pumpkin seeds.

Fats have many roles in cooking. Perhaps most important, they carry and disperse flavor throughout foods. Olive oil takes up the flavor of chili, garlic, or lemon and spreads it through the dish. Chicken breast has less flavor than dark thigh meat because it contains less fat, and modern commercial pigs, bred to be lean, make for dry and flavorless pork compared with traditional breeds. *The Bad for You Cookbook* authors want to know: "How did the fat get bred out of hogs to the point where you'd have to render three counties in Iowa to get a pound of lard?"

Fats add and retain moisture (in roasting, for example), and they keep food from sticking in frying and baking. Bakers use solid fats like butter, lard, and coconut oil to create a flaky, crumbly texture. Finally, and perhaps most mysteriously, fats contribute the inimitable quality known as "mouth feel"—think of creamy butter, silky serrano ham, or crispy skin on roast chicken. The desire for the *feel* of fat in food is universal. As anyone who has tried fat-free versions of real food knows, it has not been easy for food scientists to mimic the delectable feel of fat without real fat.

Fats, in other words, are delicious. But they are also necessary for health. Fats in the omega family are called *essential* because the body cannot make them; we must get them from foods. The brain relies on omega-3 fats; deficiency causes depression. Without fats, the body cannot absorb the fat-soluble vitamins A, D, E, and K. Fats are key to many other functions, including building cell walls, immunity, and assimilation of minerals like calcium.

Digestion is impossible without fats. The cell membrane (also made of fats) controls the muscles of the gastrointestinal tract. Fats stimulate the secretion of bile acids, which are essential for digestion. The vital role of fat in digestion is illustrated by an obscure condition called *rabbit starvation*, caused by a diet exclusively of lean protein. The term comes from Arctic explorers forced to live on lean winter game for months, and the symptoms are lethargy, nausea, diarrhea, weight loss, and eventually death. Without fat, digestion literally fails and you starve—even if you're eating plenty.

Granted, this form of malnutrition is not likely to threaten many Americans. Fat is cheap and ubiquitous—or at least industrial fats are. Today, overeating low-quality food is more often the cause of poor nutrition than starvation. So how much fat is healthy? I don't count fat grams or the percentage of calories from fat and don't recommend it. My approach is simple: I eat a variety of traditional fats and oils, and I balance rich foods with lighter ones.

However, if you would like to know how much fat people

eat and how much fat experts think we should eat, here are a few numbers. Deriving less than 20 percent of calories from fat is regarded as a low-fat diet, 30 to 40 percent moderate, and 60 percent high-fat. The extreme low-fat diet is recent, hard to follow, and nutritionally dubious. In 2006, the prestigious Women's Health Initiative trial found that low-fat diets did not prevent weight gain, heart disease, stroke, or cancer.[1] The women on the "low-fat" diet were instructed to limit fat to 20 percent of calories, but that proved impossible (or perhaps merely unpalatable). These unfortunate women, who gamely ate salads without olive oil for eight years with nothing to show for it, consumed about 29 percent of their calories from fat. That's roughly what that U.S. government recommends. The lucky women who were allowed to eat whatever they wanted (researchers call that *ad libitum,* a term I love) ate 37 percent fat, which happens to be typical of most human diets. Very high-fat diets are probably inappropriate for those of us who work at desks rather than at physical labor. Most diets—actual and recommended—are 35 to 40 percent fat. The accompanying table shows the wide range of calories from fat in diets old and new.

HOW MUCH FAT IS IN THE DIET?

Diet	*% of Calories from fat*
Nathan Pritikin and Dean Ornish	10
American Heart Association (AHA)	30
U.S. Government	30
Average U.S. diet (according to the AHA)	33
Neanderthin (based on hunter-gatherer diets)	35

Hunter-gatherers (according to Cordain's studies of 229 groups)	28–57
American cookbooks circa 1900	40*
South Beach diet, first phase	40
General Foods recommended diet in the 1930s	40
Modern Greeks	40†
American lumberjacks, circa 1911	43
Finns	39–50
Fulani, a Nigerian tribe	50*
Greenland Eskimos (rich in omega-3 fats from fish)	50
Recommended diet for infants and children up to two	50
Pacific Islanders	57*
Atkins diet, first phase	60‡

* About 50 percent saturated fat

† Mostly olive oil

‡ About 33 percent saturated fat

If You Have Only Two Minutes to Learn About Fats, Read This

WHEN I STARTED TO LEARN about the intricate chemistry of fats, it was very exciting. I studied where plant and animal fats come from and marveled at how the body makes its own fats. I wondered why the body tends to hoard polyunsaturated fats in corn oil for a rainy day, while it burns the saturated fats in butter and coconut oil quickly. Unsatisfied with the charts and tables in books, I drew my own and hung them over my desk. You can imagine my situation. I soon discovered that my friends were less fascinated with fat metabolism than I was. They asked for the essential facts on fats. Here they are.

Members of the lipid family, fats and oils (which I will call fats) consist of individual fatty acids, which may be *saturated*, *monounsaturated*, or *polyunsaturated*—terms describing their chemical structure. All fatty acids are strings of carbon atoms encircled by hydrogen atoms. When every carbon atom bonds with a hydrogen atom, the fatty acid is *saturated*. If one pair of carbon atoms forms a bond, the fatty acid is *mono*unsaturated. If two or more pairs of carbon atoms form a bond, the fatty acid is *poly*unsaturated. A carbon-hydrogen bond is known as a *saturated* or single bond. A carbon-carbon bond is called an *unsaturated* or double bond.

THE CHEMISTRY OF FATS

All fats consist of individual fatty acids made of hydrogen and carbon. Fatty acids may be saturated, monounsaturated, or polyunsaturated.

Saturated

All carbon atoms form saturated bonds with hydrogen
Example: stearic acid (beef and chocolate)

Monounsaturated

Two carbon atoms create one unsaturated bond
Example: oleic acid (olive oil and lard)

Polyunsaturated

More than one pair of carbon atoms create two or more unsaturated bonds
Example: linoleic acid (corn oil)

All the fats we eat are a blend of saturated, monounsaturated, and polyunsaturated fatty acids. Fats are identified by the *predominant* fatty acid. Beef is mostly saturated, so we call it a saturated fat—even though it contains monounsaturated and polyunsaturated fatty acids, too. Butter is mostly saturated, olive oil mostly monounsaturated, and corn oil mostly polyunsaturated. Lard is difficult to characterize because it varies with the diet of the pig, but it's about 50 percent monounsaturated, 40 percent saturated, and 10 percent polyunsaturated. Because it is 60 percent monounsaturated and polyunsaturated, lard is correctly grouped with *un*saturated fats.

An important quality of every fatty acid is its ability to withstand heat. The more saturated the fat, the more sturdy it is, because saturated bonds are stronger than unsaturated bonds. Delicate unsaturated bonds are easily damaged or oxidized by heat. When you heat a fat to the smoking point, that's a sign of damage. Unsaturated fats also spoil more quickly than saturated fats. Spoiled fats are called rancid.

Oxidized fats contribute to cancer and heart disease. According to *Science*, "Unsaturated fatty acids . . . are easily oxidized, particularly during cooking. The lipid peroxidation chain reaction (rancidity) yields a variety of mutagens . . . and carcinogens."[2] At the University of Minnesota, researchers found that repeatedly heating vegetable oils including soybean, safflower, and corn oil to frying temperature can create a toxic compound, HNE, linked to atherosclerosis, stroke, Parkinson's, Alzheimer's, and liver disease.[3] "We are, it seems, biologically primed not to eat oxidated fat," writes Margaret Visser in *Much Depends on Dinner*, "for doing so can cause diarrhea, poor growth, loss of hair, skin lesions, anorexia, emaciation, and intestinal hemorrhages." That's why it was bad news for health when fast-food restaurants stopped using saturated beef fat and palm oil, and started frying foods in rancid polyunsaturated oils.

In the kitchen, some fats are appropriate for heating, others acceptable, and some unsuitable. Heavily saturated fats (which tend to be solid at room temperature) are best for heating, monounsaturated fats are second best, and polyunsaturated fats (liquid at room temperature) are ideally used cold. Fortunately, there is a traditional fat for every culinary need. For roasting and sautéing, use butter, coconut oil, or lard, which are mostly saturated and monounsaturated. Chiefly monounsaturated oils, such as olive and macadamia nut, are the next best choice for cooking. A good blend for sautéing is half butter, half olive oil. Peanut and sesame oil, which contain more polyunsaturated fats, are less suitable for cooking but acceptable. In vinaigrettes and other cold dressings, use flaxseed, olive, or walnut oil.

THE BEST COOKING FATS

Traditional cooking fats are saturated and thus heat-stable.

Saturated	*Monounsaturated*	*Polyunsaturated*
HEAT-STABLE	MODERATELY STABLE	UNSTABLE
IDEAL FOR COOKING	ACCEPTABLE FOR MODERATE HEAT	IDEALLY USED COLD
Beef	Canola oil	Fish oil
Butter	Lard	Flaxseed oil
Coconut oil	Macadamia nut oil	Walnut oil
	Olive oil	

The body can manufacture some fats, while others, called *essential*, must be found in foods. The essential fats are polyunsaturated omega-3 (best found in fish) and omega-6 (vegetable oils). They have equally important, but opposite effects in the body. Ideally, the diet contains equal amounts of omega-3 and omega-6 fats, but the typical American eats too few omega-3 and too much of the main omega-6 fat, which leads to inflammation, obesity, diabetes, heart disease, cancer, and depression.

Omega-3 fats include alpha-linolenic acid (ALA), docosahexaenoic acid (DHA), and eicosapentaenoic acid (EPA). Flaxseed oil, grass-fed beef and butter, and pastured eggs all contain some omega-3 fats, but the best source is fish. The main omega-6 fat is linoleic acid (LA), found in grain and seed oils such as corn, safflower, and soybean oil. Once rare in the diet, the omega-6-rich oils are now ubiquitous, especially in junk food, and we eat too many.

Gamma-linolenic acid (GLA) and conjugated linoleic acid (CLA) are two omega-6 fats we should eat more of because they tend to behave like omega-3 fats in the body. In theory, the body can make GLA from the LA in corn oil, but the conversion is inhibited by many factors, so in practice the best sources are the oils of borage, black currant seed, evening primrose, and Siberian pine nuts. GLA treats premenstrual problems, reduces inflammation, dilates blood vessels, reduces clotting, and aids fat metabolism. CLA, which fights cancer and builds lean muscle, is found almost exclusively in grass-fed beef and grass-fed butter.

THE ESSENTIAL FATS

The essential fats must be eaten in the right quantities. The industrial diet contains too much LA from vegetable oils, which leads to inflammation, obesity, diabetes, and heart disease.

Omega-3	*Best source*	*Omega-6*	*Best source*
ALA	Flaxseed	LA	Corn, safflower, sunflower, and soybean oils
DHA	Fish	GLA	Black currant, borage, evening primrose, and Siberian pine nut oils
EPA	Fish	CLA	Grass-fed beef and butter

Each fat has different nutritional qualities thanks to its particular fatty acids. For example, butter contains saturated lauric acid, which fights viruses. Lard and olive oil contain monounsaturated oleic acid, which lowers LDL. Any fatty acid (such as oleic acid) is chemically identical whether it's from lard or olive oil, and has the same effect in the body.

With animal fats, the breed and especially the animal's *diet* affect fatty acid composition and nutritional value. In other words, all beef fat is not identical. Grass-fed beef contains more polyunsaturated omega-3 fat and more CLA than grain-fed beef. Grass-fed cream contains more beta-carotene, vitamin A, and CLA than cream from grain-fed cows. Lard from pigs that eat coconut contains more saturated lauric acid than lard from pigs that eat acorns.

The nutritional value of vegetable oils, on the other hand, is affected by how the oil was *processed*. Refined vegetable oils such as corn and soybean oil are pressed under high heat. Vitamin E is destroyed, and delicate polyunsaturated fats are oxidized. In extra-virgin olive oil, the antioxidants and vitamin E remain intact. Polyunsaturated oils, such as walnut and flaxseed, should be cold-pressed.

This is the most important thing about the nutrition of fats. *All the traditional fats—ideally unrefined—are healthy in moderation.* The body needs all three kinds of fats (saturated, monounsaturated, polyunsaturated) for various purposes, from pregnancy to digestion to thinking.

Aren't some fats unhealthy? Yes. It's easy to remember the bad ones: they are the industrial fats recently added to our diet. The unhealthy fats are *refined vegetable oils*, including corn, safflower, sunflower, and soybean oil, and synthetic *trans fats*. Trans fats are formed by hydrogenation, in which unsaturated oils are pelted with hydrogen atoms to make an artificially saturated fat. That's how they make firm margarine from liquid corn oil. Like natural saturated fat, hydrogenated oils are solid at room temperature and shelf-stable, which makes them useful for processed foods and baked goods. But trans fats lower HDL and cause heart disease, among other maladies. Industrial vegetable oils are unhealthy because they are too rich in omega-6 fats and because they are typically refined with heat, which makes them rancid and carcinogenic.

I've done my best to heed my friends' plea for brevity and greatly simplified the complex chemistry of fats. But the moral of the story is simple. If you're trying to remember which fats are healthy, follow this rule: *eat the foods we've eaten for thousands of years in their natural form*. If you can't find the perfect version of a food—say, 100 percent grass-fed beef—look for the next best thing. Any version of the traditional fats will be better for you than any version of the industrial fats. Those you must avoid like the proverbial Black Death.

TRADITIONAL AND INDUSTRIAL FATS
The Basics

- All the traditional fats are healthy
- The industrial diet contains too many omega-6 fats and too few omega-3 fats. This leads to obesity, diabetes, heart disease, cancer, and depression
- Trans fats lower HDL and cause heart disease, among other ills
- With animal fats, the animal's diet matters for our health
- With vegetable oils, processing matters for our health

Traditional Healthy Fats: Eat Up

ANIMAL FATS

- Fat from grass-fed cattle, sheep, bison, and other game
- Butter and cream from grass-fed cows

- Lard from pastured pigs fed a natural diet (pigs eat anything, so their diet varies)
- Egg yolks from pastured chickens, ducks, and geese
- Fish oils (preferably wild), especially cod-liver oil

VEGETABLE OILS

- Cold-pressed, extra-virgin olive oil
- Cold-pressed, unrefined flaxseed oil
- Wet-milled, unrefined coconut oil
- Cold-pressed, unrefined macadamia nut oil
- Cold-pressed, unrefined walnut oil
- Cold-pressed, unrefined sesame oil

Modern Industrial Fats: Avoid

- All hydrogenated and partially hydrogenated oils, including lard and all vegetable oils
- Corn, safflower, sunflower, and soybean oils, especially when refined or heated

How I Stopped Worrying and Learned to Love Saturated Fats

AT BONNIE SLOTNICK'S, a wonderful Greenwich Village bookshop, I was hunting for clues to the traditional American diet as if they were pottery shards, when Bonnie showed me *Twenty Lessons in Domestic Science*, a slim book billed as a "condensed home study course." It sold for two dollars in 1916, but I was happy to pay fourteen dollars. *Twenty Lessons* presents the food groups, nutritional information, recipes, and "Hints for the Housewife." "Make a business of your kitchen," it says, "and run that business as carefully as does the merchant who sells you your food." Very sensible.

All-but-forgotten frugality is not what I find curious about old nutritional primers. They illustrate just how dramatically the American diet has changed and how fast. In *Lesson No. 1: The Composition of Food Materials*, a government "Expert in Charge of Nutritional Investigations" at the U.S. Department of Agriculture provides nutritional information on meat, dairy, fish, grains, and other foods. It was the sketch of fats and oils that stood out; only five were mentioned: bacon, lard, beef suet, butter, and olive oil. In 1916, these were the fats we ate. Not anymore.

A child of my times, I once steered clear of saturated fats. Most people, and most doctors, would have regarded my diet and habits as stellar. In those days, I ate a lot of fish, vegetables, and olive oil; I was a runner and got plenty of sleep. But my digestion was poor, and I was often laid low by colds and the flu. Today my complaints are gone, I rarely get sick, and I feel great. The only change is eating saturated fats every day.

Perhaps you're like me a few years ago, and you've never heard a good word about "artery-clogging" saturated fats. Actually, they are vital to health. The most basic function of saturated fats is structural: they make up half of cell membranes. The site of all chemical activity in the body, the cell is a barrier to unwanted substances and a gateway to good ones, and the cell membrane is an extremely fine tool. A human hair is eighty thousand nanometers wide. (One million nanometers make a millimeter.) By comparison, the cell wall is tiny: only ten nanometers thick. It needs exactly the right degree of flexibility and permeability: neither too stiff nor too floppy, neither impenetrable nor too porous. Saturated fats provide stiffness, unsaturated fats flexibility.

Certain saturated fats (short- and medium-chain fatty acids) are easy to digest because they do not have to be emulsified first by bile acids, as long-chain polyunsaturated fats do. These saturated fats (in butter and coconut oil) are used directly for energy, rather than stored as fat. Saturated lauric acid in coconut oil actually increases metabolism.

Saturated fats are required for the absorption of calcium and other minerals. When the diet contains saturated fats, the body is better able to retain the vital long-chain polyunsaturated fats, such as the omega-3 fats in fish.[4] Saturated fats also build immunity by fighting harmful microbes, viruses, and other pathogens, especially in the digestive tract. Saturated lauric acid destroys the HIV virus.

Maybe you aren't convinced. Saturated fats may fight infections, but what about heart disease? Here again, I found surprises. Saturated fats lower blood levels of lipoprotein (a) (Lp(a)), which leads to clotting and atherosclerosis. Even the fats around the heart muscle are saturated.[5] They include stearic acid, found in beef and chocolate, and palmitic acid, in coconut oil, palm oil, and butter.[6] What about the "fatty" plaques in arteries that can burst and cause heart attacks? Fat is only one part, often a small one, of such plaques.[7] Moreover, only 26 percent of the fat in arterial plaques is saturated.[8] The rest is unsaturated, of which more than half is polyunsaturated.

The cholesterol theory says that eating saturated fats raises blood cholesterol in unhealthy ways. The truth is more complicated. First, about half of blood cholesterol has nothing to do with diet. Second, when you eat too much saturated fat, the body converts it to monounsaturated fat, which lowers LDL and leaves HDL alone.[9]

Furthermore, certain saturated fats (palmitic and stearic acid) have a neutral or beneficial effect on cholesterol. Forgive me for mentioning stearic acid again; perhaps I've grown partial to it because I'm fond of chocolate, but it kept turning up in my reading. Stearic acid makes a curious case study in the history of fats.

Ancel Keys, an early proponent of the cholesterol theory, made the Mediterranean diet, featuring fish, vegetables, olive oil, and red wine, famous in the 1950s and '60s. Keys developed predictive equations on diet and cholesterol. Most of his calculations, which were influential, showed that saturated fat raised cholesterol more than polyunsaturated fat, as he expected. Keys also found that stearic acid did *not* raise cholesterol, a detail he ignored. Later, other research confirmed the neutral or positive effect of stearic acid on blood cholesterol, especially the ratio of HDL to LDL. The National Research Council's report *Diet and Health* and the surgeon general's *Report on Nutrition and Health* both noted that stearic acid did not raise cholesterol. In 2005, the journal *Lipids* wrote: "Stearic acid lowers LDL cholesterol."[10]

Once the facts were in on stearic acid, did the experts tell us that the saturated fat in beef and chocolate were good for the heart? No. According to the International Food Information Council, "In light of the findings about stearic acid, some researchers recommend no longer grouping it with other saturated fats."[11] In other words, they proposed to *redefine* saturated fats rather than admit that some saturated fats don't raise cholesterol.

Diabetes is a risk factor for heart disease, and for some time, diabetics were prescribed a low-fat, high-carbohydrate diet of fruit, bread, pasta, and nonfat dairy foods. Now (sensibly) there is more emphasis on protein, but saturated fats are still taboo. The American Diabetes Association says that monounsaturated fats are best, polyunsaturated oils second-best, and saturated fats to be avoided.

Dr. Diana Schwarzbein, whose specialty is endocrine and metabolic diseases, disagrees. She found that type 2 diabetics got *worse* on a low-fat, high-carbohydrate diet. Faithful to her dietary prescriptions, her patients gained weight, their cholesterol rose, and they required more insulin, not less. Frustrated, Schwarzbein decided to experiment. When she added a little fat and protein to the menu, results were excellent. Her patients lost weight and had more energy. Their blood sugar and cholesterol fell. To her surprise, the best results were in the patients who "cheated"—they ate saturated fats and cholesterol in "real mayonnaise, real cheese, real eggs, and steak every day," she writes. In *The Schwarzbein Principle*, she describes "The Myth of Saturated Fat": "Many studies . . . vilify saturated fats . . . My clinical experience with thousands of people has shown that eating saturated fats is not the culprit! On the contrary . . . patients who have increased consumption of saturated fats (as well as all other good fats) have improved their cholesterol profiles, decreased blood pressure, and lost body fat, thereby reducing their risk of heart disease."

My own (admittedly unscientific) experience has helped convince me that saturated fats don't cause unhealthy cholesterol. As I learned more, I conducted a tiny, unintentional experiment. Gradually, I ate more saturated fat in foods like cream, chocolate, and coconut, until I was eating them every day—as I still do. After eating this way for several years, my cholesterol, HDL, LDL, triglycerides, and other signs of cardiovascular health are off-the-charts healthy by the standards of the National Cholesterol Education Program. Indeed, the more saturated fat I eat, the better the numbers look. Yet, by the logic of the cholesterol theory, I'm doing some important things wrong, and some part of me expects the numbers to look worse. But they never do.

The story is—of course—not so simple. I also do other things the experts call heart-healthy: I exercise, I don't smoke, and I eat more than my share of fruit, vegetables, olive oil, fish, dark chocolate, walnuts, and wine. I don't eat trans fats or refined vegetable oils, and I steer clear of sugar and white flour.

Mine is a balanced diet, to be sure, and the reader (or cardiologist) who favors moderation in all things might consider moderation its chief virtue. Perhaps. But I routinely eat more saturated fat than experts advise. They would not recommend eating two eggs with butter for breakfast, coconut curry for lunch, and cream in my cocoa. The medical literature has a label for people like me: *exceptions to the rule.* If saturated fats raise cholesterol, and I eat saturated fats but my cholesterol is fine, I am a "nonresponder." Or it could be that the rule is flawed.

Advice on fats is evolving. In 2004, the *American Journal of Clinical Nutrition* published a striking article. The authors called our understanding of saturated fats in particular "fragmented and biased" because research on fats had been so limited. "The approach of many mainstream investigators . . . has been narrowly focused to produce and evaluate evidence in support of the hypothesis that dietary saturated fat elevates LDL," the authors wrote. "The evidence is not strong."[12] They noted that saturated fats were "disappearing" from the food supply and asked, "Should the steps to decrease saturated fats to as low as agriculturally possible not wait until evidence clearly indicates which amounts and types of saturated fats are optimal?"[13]

Accustomed as we are to hyped headlines about miracle foods and superdrugs, this query about fats may seem innocent. Hardly. Go back and read that paragraph again. Given the conservative style of scientific literature and the heft of the conventional wisdom against saturated fats, for a prestigious journal to comment in this way is radical.

One year later, as if to answer the call for more research, along came a study of twenty-eight thousand middle-aged men and women in Malmo, Sweden.[14] Researchers looked for links between fats and mortality from heart disease and from all causes. "No deteriorating effects of high saturated fat intake were observed for either sex for any cause of death," they wrote. "Current dietary guidelines concerning fat intake are thus not supported by our observational results."

How much evidence do you need? That's up to you. But if you still fear that traditional saturated fats are trouble, my hunch is that in the next few years, more evidence in favor of butter will come your way.

Please Butter Your Carrots

IN FASHION TERMS, fats are like a string of pearls—they go with everything. The modern habit of eating chicken breasts and other lean cuts trimmed of all offending fat is new, an aberration in three million years of human history. Most people never ate protein without fat for the simple reason that in nature, protein and fat go together. In animals, fat and muscle are attached.

Eating the fat along with the protein is also frugal and efficient. Traditionally, hunters and farmers ate the whole animal, including the skin, extra fatty bits, bone marrow, brain, and rich organ meats. Contemporary human hunters, like carnivores, go for the organs and fatty parts first. Moreover, when times are good—that is, when there is plenty of food—hunters may even leave the muscle behind for scavengers. Vitamins and other nutrients in the fats and organs are simply more valuable than the lean protein.

Above all, eating protein with fat makes nutritional sense, because all food, and protein in particular, requires fat for proper digestion. As we saw earlier with "rabbit starvation," without fat in the diet, digestion fails and you starve, but not for lack of calories.

What is true of meat is true of all fat-and-protein pairs: they go together. Consider, for example, two near-perfect foods: eggs and milk. Both foods are a complete nutritional package, designed for a growing organism's exclusive nutrition, and must contain everything the body needs to assimilate the nutrients they contain. Thus the fats in the egg yolk aid digestion of the protein in the white, and lecithin in the yolk aids metabolism of its cholesterol. The butterfat in milk facilitates protein digestion, and saturated fat in particular is required to absorb the calcium. Calcium, in turn, requires vitamins A and D to be properly assimilated, and they are found only in the butterfat. Finally, vitamin A is required for production of bile salts that enable the body to digest protein. Without the butterfat, then, you don't get the best of the protein, fat-soluble vitamins, or calcium from milk. That's why I don't eat, and cannot recommend, egg white omelets and skim milk. They are low-quality, incomplete foods.

FATS GO WITH EVERYTHING

In each classic pair, fats help the body assimilate, use, or convert essential nutrients.

Fat and Protein

Roast chicken (with the skin)
Eggs (with the yolks)

Fat and Vitamins

Vitamins A, D, E, and K are fat-soluble; eat them with fat

Fat and Beta-Carotene

Buttered carrots
Collards with fatback
Spinach salad with bacon
Flank steak with arugula
Beef with broccoli

Saturated Fat and Omega-3 Fats

Fish with butter or cream sauce

Saturated Fat and Calcium

Whole milk

Yogurt, cheese, and sour cream made from whole milk

Without fats, even vegetables are less nutritious. Brightly colored vegetables are rich in antioxidant carotenoids. They go better with butter. In 2004, Iowa State University researchers who compared people eating salads with traditional or fat-free dressings found those shunning fat failed to absorb lycopene and beta-carotene, powerful antioxidants that boost immunity and fight cancer and heart disease. "Fat is necessary for the carotenoids to reach the absorptive intestinal walls," said the lead researcher, Wendy White. Lycopene is found in tomatoes and beta-carotene in orange, yellow, and green vegetables.

For vegans, who must rely entirely on vegetables for vitamin A, dressing salad with a traditional fat is even more critical. Recall that true vitamin A is found only in animal foods (especially butter, eggs, fish, and liver). The body *can* make its own vitamin A from the beta-carotene in carrots, but the conversion is costly (it requires fats and bile salts made from cholesterol) and uncertain. Babies, children, diabetics, and those with thyroid disorders make vitamin A with difficulty. Thus a person eating a strict vegan diet risks vitamin A deficiency. As Hindus and other traditional vegetarian groups know, butter and eggs are vital ingredients in vegetarian cooking.

Last but not least, the chemistry of fats can explain the long tradition of serving fish with butter and cream. Saturated fats are required to assimilate omega-3 fats, and they make omega-3 fats go farther in the body. That's the solid nutritional logic behind the delicious combinations of lobster with melted butter and Dover sole with butter sauce.

Make Mine Extra-Virgin

IN 1971, AN ITALIAN INTERNIST in her seventies named Mary Catalano was the only doctor in Buffalo who would deliver babies at home. At my mother's final prenatal checkup, Dr. Catalano, who specialized in heart disease, had an unusual question: was there olive oil at the house? The answer was yes. So, right after I was born, the doctor gently wiped my skin with olive oil. Now I wish we could ask her why. Olive oil is often used in homemade cosmetics, but I like to think of my rubdown as part of some long-lost midwifery tradition. Why not credit Dr. Catalano with my love of olive oil?

The queen of vegetable oils, olive oil is the most famous fat in the world, with a long, glorious history in cuisine and special status in many cultures. Olive oil is one of the first foods Italian babies eat, and one of the last foods offered to the dying. The evergreen olive tree grows all over the world, from Tunisia to California to Australia, and can still bear fruit at the grand age of one thousand years. Olive oil is a staple food in Greece, Italy, Portugal, and Spain, where most of the world's olive oil is produced. Its flavor is complex and varied—sometimes grassy and peppery, sometimes buttery and smooth.

Olive oil is also very good for you. It is rich in vitamin E and other powerful antioxidants called polyphenols; both nutrients prevent heart disease and cancer. By preventing oxidation, they also keep the oil itself fresh. Olive oil inhibits platelet stickiness, lowers blood pressure, and reduces inflammation. Olive oil has a good reputation with cardiologists because it is 70 percent monounsaturated oleic acid, which lowers LDL.

Olive oil is about 14 percent saturated palmitic acid (also found in palm oil, butter, and beef), which has a neutral or beneficial effect on cholesterol.[15] Palmitic acid lowers LDL.[16] Olive oil also contains about 10 percent LA, the essential omega-6 fat. But you probably don't need more LA; the industrial diet contains too much LA from vegetable oils. If you eat corn, safflower, or soybean oil, replace them with olive oil, which contains plenty of LA.

OLEIC ACID IN OLIVE OIL AND ANIMAL FATS

Food	*% of oleic acid*
Olive oil	71
Egg	50
Beef fat	48
Lard	44
Chicken fat	36
Butter	29

Healthy, delicious, and versatile in the kitchen, olive oil has never fallen out of culinary favor. It is often used cold in vinaigrettes, pesto, and other raw sauces, which protects its delicate vitamins and antioxidants, but it is also suitable for cooking at moderate temperatures because it's about 85 percent monounsaturated and saturated. Many "heart-healthy" recipes call for polyunsaturated vegetable oils such as corn or grapeseed oil for sautéeing, but olive oil is a better choice. According to *Lancet Oncology*, "The high content of the monounsaturated fat, oleic acid, is important because it is far less susceptible to oxidation than the polyunsaturated fat, linoleic acid, which predominates in sunflower oil" and other vegetable oils from grains and seeds.[17] A blend of butter and olive oil is even more heat stable because of the butter's saturated fats.

Unlike other vegetable oils, olive oil requires little processing—and for nutrition and flavor, the less the better.[18] Olive oil comes in three grades: plain, virgin, and extra-virgin. Virgin and extra-virgin oils are made in the traditional way with minimal damage to the fruit, which are simply crushed between stones without heat or chemicals. Though labor-intensive, handpicking and cold-pressing preserve delicate vitamin E and antioxidant polyphenols. According to the definition of the International Olive Oil Council, extra-virgin oil comes from the first pressing of the fruit, has no defects in taste or smell, and has acidity of 1 percent or less. Many producers have even higher standards for acidity. When olives are handpicked and cold-pressed the same day, for example, acidity is lower. The best olive oil is unfiltered to retain all its nutrients and flavor (it will be cloudy) and bottled in dark glass to shield it from oxidizing light.

Most commercial olive oil is the lowest grade—plain. It is usually labeled *olive oil,* or sometimes, confusingly, *pure* or *100 percent pure* olive oil. For this grade, the olives are picked by machine, which tends to bruise them. Bruised olives ferment and oxidize, which raises acidity and produces inferior oil.[19] The olives are pressed repeatedly with heat and subjected to chemical extraction, which diminishes nutrients and flavor. The base of plain olive oil is "lampante oil," so-called because it was once burned in lamps. Almost inedible in its crude state, it is either rancid or too acidic and must be refined to make it fit to eat. Treatments include acid washing, degumming, bleaching, and deodorization to remove foul odors.[20] The refined lampante oil is blended with virgin oil to make plain olive oil palatable.

The more olive oil is refined, the less vitamin E and antioxidants it has, and you can measure the difference: extra-virgin oil has significantly more polyphenols than lesser grades.[21] More polyphenols means better flavor and more health benefits. "High consumption of extra virgin olive oils, which are particularly rich in these phenolic antioxidants . . . should afford considerable protection against cancer (colon, breast, skin), coronary heart disease, and ageing by inhibiting oxidative stress," say antioxidant experts.[22] Women who eat olive oil (and fruits and vegetables) significantly reduce the risk of breast cancer, while eating margarine increases it.[23]

How, exactly, does olive oil fight heart disease and cancer? Oxidized LDL is a cause of heart disease. Polyphenols inhibit oxidation of LDL, and the more the better.[24] Polyphenols may also stimulate antioxidant enzymes and increase HDL. Another antioxidant in extra-virgin oil, squalene, fights skin cancer. Still other antioxidants called lignans inhibit cell growth in cancers of the skin, breast, colon, and lung.

To reap all the flavor and health benefits of olive oil, buy the best oil you can afford, ideally extra-virgin, cold-pressed, and organic. I use extra-virgin oil, even for cooking. When you heat extra-virgin oil, antioxidants counter the damage to the delicate vitamin E and unsaturated fats. If that's too expensive, use virgin oil for frying and extra-virgin for cold dressings. Beware of "light" olive oil. It's a marketing gimmick to make you think it has fewer calories. Refined to remove color and scent, it lacks the flavor and antioxidants of extra-virgin oil. Store olive oil away from heat and light.

Most olive oils, including better-quality brands, are blends of different crops, to ensure consistent flavor and quality, not unlike wine blended from different grape harvests. The very best olive oils, again like wines, are estate bottled, which typically means the olives from one harvest were pressed and bottled where they were grown. Fancy estate oils are often seasonal and usually quite delicious. But for me, at least, they're a rare treat. I use a lot of olive oil, so I watch my budget.

My Opinion of the Minor Vegetable Oils

WHAT OIL IS BEST FOR SAUTÉING? When I talk with people about fats, this is one of the most common questions they ask me. The short answer: not polyunsaturated vegetable oils such as corn, safflower, sunflower, and soybean oil. Those fats are too delicate. When heated, they oxidize and become rancid and carcinogenic. The best cooking fats are mostly saturated, such as butter, beef, and coconut oil. Second best are the mostly monounsaturated fats, such as lard, macadamia nut oil, and olive oil.

These answers, unfortunately, don't satisfy most people. They might regard olive oil as too expensive for everyday cooking. Often they're looking for a "neutral" flavor. The bland taste of lard makes it a great platform for flavors sweet and savory—one reason it's perfect for pie crust. However, it seems that many people are not ready to start frying chicken in lard, even though good cooks all over the world do just that. Olive oil, butter, and coconut oil do have pronounced flavors. I love the scent, flavor, and feel of coconut oil, but usually I save it for certain dishes like Sri Lankan fish curry. Coconut oil does not flatter asparagus or new potatoes.

The goal of a "neutral" flavor is tricky anyway—perhaps even futile. Fats, more than any other food, are aromatic. They not only *have* flavor but also *carry* flavors on the palate. Having tasted many fats, I've concluded there is no such thing as a flavorless fat. Butter tastes like cream, olive oil like olives, corn oil like corn. That's why many oils (including avocado, olive, corn, and coconut) are refined, bleached, or deodorized—to strip them of scent and flavor. The result is a bland fat, to be sure, but with unhappy results, in every case, for the nutrients in the natural version.

It may be best to forget the quest for a "neutral" flavor. Fats are assertive; for that reason they lend character to whole cuisines.

Middle Eastern dishes call for frying many foods in lamb fat. Most Americans would call that a very strong flavor; lamb colors all the dishes, in the same way olive oil leaves its mark on the cuisine of Greece, where even desserts are made with the herbaceous oil. We may regard olive oil as somehow more neutral tasting than lamb fat, so redolent of lanolin, but that's merely a matter of taste and familiarity.

My advice is to treat fats as you would any other ingredient: choose the feel and the flavor to match the dish. As I've mentioned, I mostly use butter and olive oil, or a combination, for sautéing and roasting. For certain dishes, like roasted red peppers, I use only olive oil, and I simply don't worry about the few polyunsaturated fats it contains. But it is true that heating any unsaturated oil is less than ideal. Sometimes I blanch or steam vegetables and add the olive oil after cooking, which has the added virtue of showcasing the flavor of relatively expensive extra-virgin oil.

Even after I confess to heating olive oil and reveal my (unoriginal) olive oil-and-butter blend secret, people still want to know about neutral vegetable oils for sautéing, frying, and dressing salads. There are many culinary vegetable and nut oils, from Brazil nut to grapeseed to pecan; you will have to find your favorites. (See the accompanying sidebar for a few vegetable oils I might use—or wouldn't disapprove of, anyway—other than olive and coconut oil.)

A FEW OTHER VEGETABLE OILS

Acceptable for Cooking

- Macadamia nut oil is about 85 percent monounsaturated, which makes it suitable for cooking, though I prefer it cold. Buttery and nutty, it has a lovely flavor, but it's not cheap.
- Peanut oil is 46 percent monounsaturated oleic acid, 31

percent polyunsaturated LA, and about 17 percent saturated. Because it's about 60 percent monounsaturated and saturated, it's fine for cooking, if the flavor suits you. Don't buy hydrogenated oil.

- Sesame oil is 43 percent polyunsaturated LA, 41 percent monounsaturated, and 15 percent saturated. It's suitable for cooking, but the flavor is hardly neutral, especially toasted oil. Its unique antioxidants, including sesamin, are *not* destroyed by heat like most antioxidants; they protect the polyunsaturated fats. In Chinese cooking, sesame oil is typically used cold in salads or added after cooking.

Best Used Cold

- Flaxseed oil comes from linseed. Ground flaxseed has been a traditional food and medicine in the Mediterranean region and Africa for thousands of years. It's the best plant source of omega-3 ALA (60 percent), which the body uses to make DHA and EPA. Flaxseed oil has a distinctive herbaceous, woody flavor. A blend of flaxseed and olive oil in vinaigrette is a good way to slip omega-3 fats to vegetarians and people who don't eat enough fish. ALA is very sensitive to light and heat. Keep flaxseed oil in the fridge.
- Grapeseed oil is about 70 percent polyunsaturated LA and rich in heat-sensitive vitamin E, which makes it a poor frying fat. I don't use it, mostly because it's so rich in omega-6 fats, but people like it for its neutral flavor.
- Walnut oil is about 54 percent polyunsaturated LA. It also contains about 12 percent omega-3 ALA. Highly unsaturated, walnut oil should be cold-pressed, kept cold, and used cold. It has a pronounced, tannic flavor I happen to love, and I use it often in salad dressing, sometimes with roasted walnuts.

What about the common vegetable oils grown in the American heartland, including corn, safflower, sunflower, and soybean oil? I don't use, or recommend, any of the modern vegetable oils. They're rich in polyunsaturated omega-6 LA (too delicate for heat), and most Americans eat far too many omega-6 fats already. They also lower HDL. Fran McCullough has a sensible take on high-oleic acid sunflower oil in *Good Fat*: "If you desperately need a flavorless oil that's not light [refined] olive oil, this is your best candidate, as long as it's expeller-pressed (cold-pressed, without high heat), not hydrogenated, and stored carefully. Still, this is a fragile oil with no particular health benefits beyond its high-oleic additive."[25]

Other vegetable oils mentioned here—sesame, peanut, and grapeseed—are also fairly rich in omega-6 LA. That's one reason I seldom use them, but I also prefer other oils. If you don't eat corn, safflower, sunflower, or soybean oil, a little sesame or peanut oil, if that's what you prefer for a broccoli stir-fry, won't do any harm.

Coconut Oil Is Good for You

IN THE NINETEENTH CENTURY, coconut oil was common in baked goods, from cookies to crackers. A saturated fat like coconut oil is ideal for baking because it's stable when heated, remains solid at room temperature (which makes things flaky), and has a long shelf life. Cookie companies and home bakers alike used it. An 1896 ad for "pure and wholesome cocoanut butter" recommended it in place of lard and butter and boasted endorsements from chefs and doctors.

By the middle of the twentieth century, coconut had all but disappeared from the American diet. What happened? It was a commercial battle over what fat would be used in baked goods, and the competitors were domestic vegetable oils and imported tropical oils, including palm and coconut oil. As the two industries fought for market share, nutrition experts threw the knockout punch: the idea that saturated fats cause heart disease. Coconut oil imports never recovered.

Today, most commercial baked goods are made with another solid and shelf-stable fat: hydrogenated vegetable oil. That turned out badly; now we know that trans fats cause heart disease. Meanwhile, coconut oil turns out to be innocent of the cholesterol charges, with other virtues in the bargain.

The coconut palm tree grows in the tropics and subtropics, including Asia, India, Africa, and Latin America, where the milk, flesh, and oil of the coconut fruit are used in a variety of dishes, from drinks to soups and sauces. Coconut flesh contains fiber, fat, vitamins B, C, and E, and calcium, magnesium, iron, zinc, and potassium. Coconut oil is a folk remedy in many cultures, from the Philippines to Sri Lanka. Polynesians, who eat coconut and coconut oil every day, call it the "Tree of Life."

Like all saturated fats, coconut oil is solid at room temperature; it turns soft at about seventy-six degrees Fahrenheit. The oil is rich (64 percent) in medium-chain saturated fatty acids, which have unusual properties. The main fat (49 percent) is lauric acid, an antimicrobial, antifungal, and antiviral fatty acid all but unique to coconut oil and breast milk. Lauric acid kills fat-coated viruses, including HIV, measles, herpes, influenza, leukemia, hepatitis C, Epstein-Barr, and bacteria, such as *Listeria*, *Helicobacter pylori*, and strep.[26] Monolaurin, an agent the body makes from lauric acid, fights the herpes and cytomegalovirus viruses.[27]

The medium-chain fats in coconut oil don't need to be emulsified by bile acids before they are digested, as long-chain polyunsaturated fats do. Thus the body burns coconut oil more quickly than long-chain polyunsaturated fats like soybean oil, which it tends to store for later. For this reason, lauric acid is easy to digest, and for decades doctors have fed coconut oil to patients unable to digest polyunsaturated fats.[28]

Medium-chain fats can also aid weight loss. Ultimately, of course, the most important thing is how much energy you consume and spend, but metabolism is more subtle than that. For example, lean protein has a higher "thermic effect" than fat or carbohydrate; that means it gives metabolism a boost. Lauric acid has a similar effect. A large number of studies in both animals and people show that coconut oil, when compared with polyunsaturated fats, enhances weight loss.[29]

What about heart disease? In the 1960s, Dr. Ian Prior, director of epidemiology at Wellington Hospital in New Zealand, studied all twenty-five hundred people on the South Pacific islands Pukapuka and Tokelau. Coconut was the bulk of the diet, appearing at every meal as a drink, vegetable, dessert, or cooking oil. They ate pork, poultry, seafood, and produce, too, but the striking thing about their diet is the large amount of fat and saturated fat. On Tokelau, 57 percent of calories came from fat, about half of it saturated. On Pukapuka, they ate sixty-three grams of saturated fat daily and seven grams of unsaturated fat. Yet all the islanders were lean and healthy, with no signs of unhealthy cholesterol, atherosclerosis, or heart disease.

Then, by chance, nature presented an experiment. When crop failure forced Tokelau islanders to move to New Zealand, they ate less coconut oil, less fat, half as much saturated fat, and more polyunsaturated oils than at home. Good for the heart, right? But in 1981, Prior found his subjects living in New Zealand in *worse* health: the immigrants had higher cholesterol, higher LDL, and lower HDL.[30] "The more an Islander takes on the ways of the West, the more prone he is to succumb to our degenerative diseases," Prior said.

In the last thirty years, a number of studies have cleared coconut oil of any role in heart disease, and recent research confirms those findings.[31] In 2002, researchers fed people seventy to eighty grams of medium-chain fats or vegetable oils daily and found no differences in total cholesterol, VLDL, LDL, or HDL, or triglycerides.[32] Other researchers who fed medium-chain fats to rats stated bluntly, "The lipid [fats] theory of arteriosclerosis is rejected." They noted that Sri Lanka, where coconut oil is the main fat, had low mortality from heart disease.[33]

Coconut oil even improves the all-important ratio of HDL and LDL.[34] A study of Malaysians who ate palm, coconut, or corn oil for five weeks found that coconut oil increased HDL, improving the ratio.[35] In the same study, saturated palmitic acid (found in another tropical fat, palm oil) lowered total cholesterol and LDL.

How, then, did coconut oil get a bad reputation? Partly because we misunderstood cholesterol. We used to think that any fat that raised *total* cholesterol, as coconut oil can, was unhealthy, but now we know that total cholesterol is a poor predictor of heart disease and that raising HDL is good. Moreover, hydrogenated coconut oil was used in some studies. In 1996, the lipids expert Mary Enig explained that hydrogenation raises cholesterol: "Problems for coconut oil started four decades ago when researchers fed animals hydrogenated coconut oil purposefully altered to make it devoid of essential fatty acids. Animals fed hydrogenated coconut oil (as the only fat) became essential fatty acid-deficient; their cholesterol levels increased. Diets that cause an essential fatty acid deficiency always produce an increase in cholesterol."[36]

In 2001, researchers reported that partially hydrogenated soybean oil was worse than coconut oil. "Epidemiological and experimental studies suggest that trans fatty acids increase risk more than do saturates because [trans fats] lower HDL," they wrote. "Solid fats rich in lauric acids, such as tropical fats, appear to be preferable to trans fats in food manufacturing, where hard fats are indispensable."[37]

Big food companies may not be rushing to put coconut oil back in crackers, but you can put fresh coconut, dried flakes, and coconut milk, cream, and oil in cookies, soups and curries. Many people take a spoonful of coconut oil daily to aid weight loss and boost immunity.

Coconut oil comes in three unofficial grades. The best is unrefined or virgin oil, made by shredding and cold-pressing coconut flesh while it is moist, a process called *wet milling*. The meat, milk, and oil are fermented for at least twenty-four hours while the water and oil separate. Finally, the oil is gently heated to remove moisture and filtered. Virgin oil has the lovely flavor and scent of coconut.

The second-best coconut oil is expeller-pressed and gently deodorized to remove scent and flavor; it's a good choice if you eat coconut oil for health but don't care for the flavor. Industrial coconut oil is made by extracting oil from *copra*, or dry coconut meat. To make it edible, the oil is refined, bleached, and deodorized, which destroys vitamins, scent, and flavor.

I buy virgin coconut oil and cream, along with wonderful soap and moisturizer, from a cooperative of small growers in the Philippines called Tropical Traditions. You can also find good brands of virgin coconut oil in whole foods shops, good groceries, and Asian shops. Virgin coconut oil isn't cheap, but I don't use it every day, a little goes a long way, and it keeps for two years without refrigeration. Canned coconut milk is less expensive. I like to have a couple of cans in the cupboard for making a simple, creamy soup made of equal parts chicken stock and coconut milk, with sautéed ginger and cayenne. Everyone loves it.

7

Industrial Fats

How the Margarine Makers Outfoxed the Dairy Farmers

THE ADVICE TO REPLACE BUTTER with margarine containing trans fats constituted a radical dietary experiment. Trans fats are created when oil is hydrogenated. That's when unsaturated oil is blasted with hydrogen atoms, a form of artificial saturation that makes the liquid oil solid, like natural saturated fats. But the similarity between trans fats and traditional saturated fats ends there. Trans fats are new and dangerous. Traditional diets contain healthy saturated fats from both plants (like coconut) and animals (butter), but until the twentieth century, no one ate trans fats, and now we know they cause heart disease.[1]

Hydrogenated vegetable oils are widely used in cakes, cookies, donuts, chips, and crackers, for the same reason food companies once used coconut oil: they're solid, heat-stable, and don't spoil easily. Though it's possible to hydrogenate any fat that is not fully saturated (such as lard, which is about 60 percent unsaturated), most hydrogenated oils are made from polyunsaturated vegetable oils such as canola, corn, and soybean. In a moment we'll come back to trans fats, but first, let's look at margarine, the mother of hydrogenated oils.

In the nineteenth century, a patriotic French chemist, who had already earned gold medals for making bread with less flour, invented margarine. A cattle plague having recently devastated European herds, "butter was difficult to get and expensive," writes Margaret Visser in *Much Depends on Dinner*. Napoleon III offered a prize for the invention of a cheaper substitute for butter. Tinkering on the imperial farm in Vincennes, Hippolyte Mège-Mouriès won the prize in 1869, for his blend of beef fat and sheep stomach, with added milk for flavor.

This inexpensive, solid fat—known in English as oleomargarine—was taken up by the Dutch and English poor, who, like other European peasants, couldn't afford butter. When the first U.S. oleomargarine plant opened in Manhattan in the 1870s, Americans, blessed with ample green pastures, were in a better position: there was still plenty of butter to be had. Although the Chicago-based meatpacking industry doggedly promoted oleomargarine as a cheaper substitute for butter, the unappealing white blocks were not an overnight success with American cooks.

Dairy farmers, however, rightly saw a long-term commercial threat from this less expensive upstart and began to lobby furiously for laws to restrict margarine sales. For example, they stopped it from ever being called "butter." Margarine makers fought back, proposing, quite sensibly, to dye margarine yellow to make it look like butter. Color had always been the buyer's clue to butter quality. Grass-fed butter, rich in vitamin A, is yellow, while butter from grain-fed cows is white.

With the help of friendly politicians, dairy farmers put a stop to yellow dye, and five states with dairy muscle even forced margarine makers to dye it pink, apparently intending to make it look ridiculous. Undeterred, margarine makers responded by selling the white blocks with a packet of yellow dye to mix in at home. This, presumably, would fool the family—if not the cook.

"On the whole," writes Visser, "the producers of butter fought a very dirty fight." But in vain. After a series of skirmishes, the dairy industry gradually lost clout, while the power of margarine manufacturers grew. By 1950, President Harry Truman had repealed the last of the antimargarine laws, and punishing taxes on margarine were lifted. The modern margarine business was off and running.

Meanwhile, a revolutionary method for making solid fats was soon to transform the margarine industry, according to the food writer Linda Joyce Forristal, who is famous for lard pie crusts and better known as Mother Linda.[2] In the late 1890s, the soap and candle company Proctor & Gamble was fed up with the high price of lard and tallow—the market was controlled by the powerful meatpacking industry—and began to look for alternatives. It settled on cottonseed oil and in classic capitalist fashion soon owned eight cottonseed plants in Mississippi, the better to secure its supply. In 1907, company scientists figured out how to make liquid oil solid by firing it with hydrogen. "Mindful that electrification was forcing the candle business into decline, P&G looked for other markets for their new product," explains Forristal. "Since hydrogenated cottonseed oil resembled lard, why not sell it as a food?"

Introduced in 1911, the new product was presented as healthier, cheaper, and cleaner than butter and lard. Proctor & Gamble promoted the spreadable white vegetable fat in women's magazines and gave away a cookbook with 615 recipes calling for its brand name: Crisco. The marketing department spent time on Jewish cooks in particular. Crisco made it easier to keep kosher because it was like butter but could be eaten with meats, and it was also a substitute for lard.

Then, in the 1950s, came another fillip for plucky, can't-knock-me-down margarine: official advice that saturated fats were unhealthy. The makers of Crisco and the vegetable oil industry worked to spread the word that animal fats caused heart disease.

Food companies and restaurants came under pressure to stop using coconut oil, butter, and lard. With hydrogenation, the vegetable oil industry could offer what seemed to be the ideal fat: polyunsaturated, yet solid and shelf-stable. And that, dear reader, is how trans fats pushed lard and butter out of American kitchens.

A RECIPE FOR MARGARINE

Begin with a polyunsaturated, liquid vegetable oil rancid from extraction under high heat. Any oil will do, but about 85 percent of hydrogenated oils are soybean. Mix with tiny metal particles, usually nickel oxide. In a high-pressure, high-temperature reactor, shoot hydrogen atoms at the unsaturated carbon bonds. Add soaplike emulsifiers and starch to make it soft and creamy. Steam to remove foul odors, bleach away the gray color, dye it yellow, and add artificial flavors. If you prefer real food, but you like a soft spread, try this idea from Fran McCullough: mix equal parts room-temperature butter and olive oil until creamy. Add unrefined salt to taste.

As we now know, the experiment with margarine ended badly, spectacularly so. Trans fats wreak havoc all over the body, and for a long time, these dangerous fats were hard to detect. Nutrition labels listed saturated and unsaturated fats, but the careful consumer had to read the ingredient list for "hydrogenated" or "partially hydrogenated" oils to avoid trans fats. In 2006, things got easier, when the FDA required food labels to list trans fats. "The minute it goes on the label, it's out of the food supply," said Dr. Marion Nestle, a professor at New York University. "That's how food policy is done in this country."

How Fake Butter Causes Heart Disease

> [Trans fats are the] biggest food-processing disaster in U.S. history . . . In Europe [food companies] hired chemists and took trans fats out . . . In the United States, they hired lawyers and public relations people.
>
> —Professor Walter Willett,
> Harvard School of Public Health

IN THE LAST CENTURY, the American diet changed radically, but *how* it changed might surprise you. Given that heart disease began to be a problem around 1950, you might guess that we eat more saturated fats than in 1900. But in fact we eat less butter, lard, and beef and vastly more polyunsaturated oils now. In another way, however, the assumption that we eat more "artery-clogging" saturated fats is dead right: today we eat an industrial saturated fat that didn't exist in 1900. Before World War II, Americans ate about 12 grams of trans fats daily, by 1985 as much as 40 grams.[3] Since the 1970s, Americans have eaten roughly twice as much margarine as butter. For a major cause of heart disease, look no farther. Lard and butter "aren't public enemy No. 1 anymore," says Dr. Frank Hu of the Harvard School of Public Health. That designation now belongs to trans fats.

According to Dr. Walter Willett at Harvard, trans fats cause up to one hundred thousand premature deaths annually from heart disease.[4] Compared with saturated fat, trans fats raise triglycerides, reduce blood vessel function, and raise lipoprotein (a) (Lp(a)), which causes clots and atherosclerosis.[5] They raise LDL and reduce HDL. Willett says trans fats are twice as bad for the HDL/LDL ratio as saturated fats. Even experts who are cautious about saturated fat agree that butter is better.

I find it dismaying that the dangers of trans fats were known for sixty years. Weston Price cited 1943 research that butter was better than hydrogenated cottonseed oil. In the 1950s, researchers guessed that hydrogenated vegetable oil led to heart disease.[6] Ancel Keys, the proponent of monounsaturated fat, showed in 1961 that hydrogenated corn oil raised triglycerides more than butter.[7] Year after year, the bad news piled up.

One dogged researcher, Mary Enig, helped to get the word out. The author of *Know Your Fats*, Enig waged an often lonely battle. I'm afraid her efforts were not always welcomed with bouquets of roses. In 1978, Enig wrote a scientific paper challenging a government report blaming saturated fat for cancer, in which she pointed out that the data actually showed a link with trans fats. Not long after, "two guys from the Institute of Shortening and Edible Oils—the trans fat lobby, basically—visited me, and boy, were they angry," Enig told *Gourmet* magazine.[8] "They said they'd been keeping a careful watch to prevent articles like mine from coming out and didn't know how this horse had gotten out of the barn."

The stakes were high. "We spent lots of time, and lots of money and energy, refuting this work," said Dr. Lars Wiederman, who once worked for the American Soybean Association. "Protecting trans fats from the taint of negative scientific findings was our charge."

TRANS FATS: UNSAFE AT ANY MEAL

- Lower HDL
- Raise LDL
- Raise Lp(a), which promotes atherosclerosis and clotting
- Reduce blood vessel function
- Promote obesity, diabetes, and hypertension
- Alter fat cell size and number

- Reduce cream in breast milk
- Reduce fertility and correlate with low birth weight
- Increase asthma
- Reduce immune response
- Interfere with the conversion and use of DHA and EPA
- Disrupt enzymes that metabolize carcinogens and drugs
- Damage cell membranes
- Create free radicals

Main source: Enig Associates.

At Harvard, meanwhile, Willett and his colleagues produced definitive studies on trans fats, providing data that proved crucial in convincing the government that trans fats were unsafe. In 1999, Willett described how the food industry had tried to delay the guilty verdict.

> Food manufacturers use partial hydrogenation of vegetable oil to destroy some fatty acids, such as linolenic and linoleic acid, which tend to oxidize, causing fat to become rancid. Commercial production of partially hydrogenated fats began in the early 20th century and increased steadily until about the 1960s as processed vegetable fats displaced animal fats in the diet. Lower cost was the initial motivation, but health benefits were later claimed for margarine as a replacement for butter . . . Trans fats [are] associated with an increased risk of coronary heart disease. In response to these reports, a 1995 review sponsored by the food industry concluded that the evidence was insufficient to take action and further research was needed.[9]

Fortunately for the public, researchers did carry on. Unfortunately for the trans fat lobby, the news got worse. At last, official word came from the National Academy of Sciences, which announced in 2002 that trans fats have "no known health benefits" and no level of consumption is safe.[10]

As the list in the preceding sidebar shows, trans fats do a lot of damage in addition to causing heart disease. Recall that all of your cell walls are made of fat. Like natural fats, trans fats enter the tissues and become part of the cell membrane, where, unlike natural fats, they disrupt every cellular activity, from metabolism to immunity. Hundreds of thousands of Americans are walking around with cell walls made of trans fats, which have no place in the diet or the body. The deadly effects of industrial trans fats will be with us for some time. The sooner we ban trans fats—as Denmark has—the better.[11]

Why I Don't Eat Corn, Soybean, or Sunflower Oil

SINCE THE 1970S, experts have urged us to eat less fat and to replace saturated fats with polyunsaturated oils. Did Americans do as they were told? Yes and no. In 2000, we ignored official advice and ate more total fat than before. In the low-fat era, this may be surprising; larger portions of junk foods and plain old gluttony probably played a part. We did eat more vegetable oils, as instructed. Perhaps we were simply obedient and used more vegetable oils in cooking, but I suspect Americans didn't always choose the polyunsaturated oils now ubiquitous in cookies, crackers, and other processed foods. Sometimes, the food supply changes, not only without our say-so, but without our being the wiser. In this case, cheap vegetable oils (often hydrogenated) were the ingredient the food industry chose, and those were the fats we got.

U.S. CONSUMPTION OF FATS AND OILS

	Pounds per person per year	
	1991	*2000*
Total fat	65.5	74.6
Butter	4.3	4.5
Margarine	10.6	8.3
Salad and cooking oils	26.7	33.7

Source: USDA Agricultural Statistics, 2003.

Perhaps you're thinking what I thought when I first saw these figures: vegetable oils are a good source of omega-6 linoleic acid (LA), one of the essential fats. What's wrong with that? In modest amounts, nothing. But we eat far too many. The balance between the two essential fats, omega-3 and omega-6, is out of whack. We should eat equal amounts, but the industrial diet has about twenty times more omega-6 than omega-3 fats. For three million years, no human ate like that.

The flood of omega-6 fats comes from the American heartland, once known for rippling wheat fields. This lovely image is outdated. Today the bread basket is more like an oil field, studded with rigs spewing soybean and corn oil. (And corn syrup and starch. The writer Michael Pollan calls corn "the keystone species of the industrial food system.")[12] The heartland oils are fountains of omega-6 fats. Soybean oil is 53 percent omega-6, corn 57 percent, sunflower 68 percent, and safflower 78 percent. Corn oil contains sixty times more omega-6 than omega-3 fats. In safflower oil, the ratio is 77:1. That's a long way from the ideal ratio of 1:1.

"The current Western diet is very high in omega-6 fats because of the indiscriminate recommendation to substitute omega-6 fats for saturated fats to lower serum cholesterol," says Dr. Artemis

Simopoulos, author of *The Omega Diet*. Industrial farming has made things worse: "Intake of omega-3 fats is much lower today because of the decrease in fish consumption and the industrial production of animal feeds rich in grains containing omega-6 fats, leading to production of meat rich in omega-6 and poor in omega-3 fats. The same is true for cultured fish and eggs."[13]

What's wrong with eating too many omega-6 fats? From the omega fats, the body makes chemicals called eicosanoids, hormone-like agents with far-reaching effects on metabolism, inflammation, immunity, fertility, blood pressure, skin, vision, and mood. "Eicosanoids are involved from the top of the head in the brain to the nerves at the bottom of the feet and everywhere in between," writes Kenneth Broughton, a professor of nutrition at the University of Wyoming.[14]

Omega-3 and omega-6 eicosanoids play opposite and equally vital roles. Omega-3 eicosanoids are anti-inflammatory and calming, for example, while omega-6 eicosanoids are inflammatory and reactive. Late in pregnancy, omega-6 eicosanoids prompt labor to begin and omega-3 fats prevent premature birth. Omega-6 agents suppress, and omega-3 agents promote, ovulation.[15] By promoting clotting, omega-6 eicosanoids stop you from bleeding to death from a small cut. Omega-3 eicosanoids, on the other hand, thin the blood, which helps prevent heart attack and stroke. (There is one notable exception: the omega-6 fat GLA tends to behave more like an omega-3, fighting inflammation and heart disease. GLA is in the oils of black currant, borage, evening primrose, and Siberian pine nut.)

Imagine a body dominated by omega-6 eicosanoids; symptoms would include inflammation, obesity, insulin resistance, premature labor, infertility, blood clots, and depression. As for heart disease, omega-6 eicosanoids are trouble. They promote inflammation, constrict blood vessels, and encourage platelet stickiness and clotting. Oxidized omega-6 fats lead to oxidized LDL, which causes atherosclerosis.[16]

Omega-6 fats are the key to a mystery scientists dubbed the "Israeli Paradox." In 1996, researchers noted that Israeli Jews followed the recommended diet for preventing obesity, diabetes, and heart disease. They ate fewer calories, more carbohydrates, less fat, less saturated fat, and more polyunsaturated vegetable oils than Americans. In fact, their diet closely resembled the USDA food pyramid, including generous amounts of fruit and vegetables. Notably, they ate more omega-6 fats than any group in the world. The reward for this dietary discipline? Higher rates of obesity and diabetes than Americans and similar rates of heart disease. "Rather than being beneficial," said researchers, "high omega-6 polyunsaturated fatty acid diets may have some long-term side effects within the cluster of hyperinsulinemia, atherosclerosis, and tumorigenesis."[17] In plain words, omega-6 fats lead to diabetes, heart disease, and cancer. There is strong evidence that omega-6 fats make cancer cells grow faster.[18]

FAT CONSUMPTION IN U.S. AND ISRAELI POPULATIONS

Israelis eat less fat and more polyunsaturated oils than Americans, yet they have higher rates of obesity and diabetes and similar rates of heart disease. Scientists blame excess omega-6 LA.

	Americans	*Israelis*
Calories (per day)	3,455	2,999
Calories from fat (%)	43.9	32.7
Ratio of polyunsaturated to saturated fat	0.63	1.6
Calories from carbohydrates (%)	44	53.3

Source: Susan Allport, "The Skinny on Fat," *Gastronomica* 3, no. 1 (2003): 28–36.

Americans are on the same unhealthy track. We eat too many vegetable oils, too few natural saturated fats, and too many refined carbohydrates, which raise triglycerides. This is new. When our ancestors ate grains and omega-6 fats, they came from whole foods: leafy plants, whole wheat, and corn. Native Americans rarely, if ever, ate pure corn oil. They ate the whole corn kernel: bran, carbohydrate, oil, and all. Corn was ground slowly between stones, leaving its unsaturated fats and antioxidant vitamin E intact. People ate whole grains and fresh, unrefined oils.

Industrial vegetable oil processing, by contrast, removes flavor and nutrients. Grain, beans, and seeds are crushed under high heat and extracted with chemical solvents like hexane, which is then boiled off. They may be bleached, refined, and deodorized. All this damages the polyunsaturated fats, destroys vitamin E, and creates free radicals.

Modern vegetable oils are not my idea of real food. Corn, safflower, soybean, and sunflower oil have little flavor, which is reason enough not to eat them. Moreover, they don't contain any important nutrient that I can't find in some other traditional food. You can get all the vitamin E you need from almonds, avocados, and whole grains, and more than enough omega-6 fats from olive oil.

I Am Not Convinced by Canola

IN THE ANNALS OF OILS, canola oil is worth a little detour, because it is a unique vegetable oil and much celebrated by advocates of the "heart healthy" diet. Perhaps the most famous modern vegetable oil, canola is made from rapeseed, a member of the genus *Brassica*, which includes broccoli and cabbage. Unusually for a seed oil, it's rich in monounsaturated fat, with some omega-3 fats, too. In recent years, Americans have added huge amounts of canola oil to their diets. In 1992, the United States imported 381,000 metric tons of canola oil; in 2001, 540,000 tons came in.

Traditional rapeseed oil has a long history of culinary use in China and India, where the seeds were ground between stones and they used the oil fresh, probably in relatively small quantities, given the slow method of making oil. Unfortunately, much of the fat (about 50 percent) in rapeseed is erucic acid, which causes lesions on the heart. Scientists have long been aware of the erucic acid problem, and in the 1970s they bred a new rapeseed oil low in erucic acid. They called it canola, for Canadian oil.

This new rapeseed oil is typically about 60 percent monounsaturated oleic acid, 20 percent polyunsaturated omega-6, 10 percent polyunsaturated omega-3, and most of the rest is saturated. With this combination of fats, canola oil was promoted as good for the heart and sales grew quickly. Official dietary advice and cookbooks were key to the campaign, with many recipes calling for heart-friendly monounsaturated canola oil to lower cholesterol. In 1985, canola oil won GRAS status—Generally Recognized as Safe—from the FDA. Highly coveted, GRAS means that a company doesn't have to prove an ingredient is safe each time it is added to foods.

However, canola oil isn't perfect. The ratio of omega-6 to omega-3 fats in canola oil (2:1) is not ideal—but it's not terrible, either. As we've seen, an equal amount of omega-6 and omega-3 fats is best. Like other modern vegetable oils, most canola oil is refined under heat and pressure, which damages its omega-3 fats. Because canola oil is more easily hydrogenated than some vegetable oils, it is often used in processed foods. Finally, much of the low-erucic acid canola oil crop is genetically engineered.

It's difficult to find neutral information on canola. Its fans and critics are equally firm. For obvious reasons, there are no long-term studies: low-erucic acid canola oil is a relatively new food. Many of the alarming claims making the rounds are probably overstated, and I won't repeat them here. However, animal studies have linked canola oil with reduced platelet count, shorter life span, and greater need for vitamin E. The United States and Canada do not permit canola oil to be used in infant formula because it retards growth in animals. In one human study, canola oil raised triglycerides (fats that are part of the "total cholesterol" number) while saturated fats lowered triglycerides.[19]

Despite these caveats, many nutritionists are enthusiastic about canola oil for its monounsaturated fats. Loren Cordain, the expert on Stone Age diets, favors canola oil, even though it is a very modern food. "There is no credible scientific evidence showing that canola oil is harmful to humans," he says.

I never use canola oil, largely because I have no reason to. For flavor, health, and cooking, I simply prefer other fats. The flavor of canola oil is nothing special. Wild salmon and flaxseed oil are a far better source of omega-3 fats, and olive and macadamia nut oil are more delicious sources of monounsaturated fats. For sautéing and roasting, I prefer to use olive oil and butter, and for baking, butter or lard.

If you do use canola oil, recall the general rule for unsaturated fats: buy cold-pressed, unrefined oil and heat it gently, never to the smoking point. If you would like to avoid genetically engineered rapeseed, look for certified organic oil.

8

Other Real Foods

The Abominable Egg White Omelet

AS LONG AS I CAN REMEMBER, my mother has eaten her breakfast in the late morning. When she comes in hungry from watering the greenhouse, the squash pick, or any number of early morning jobs, breakfast is two eggs in butter, yolks runny, toast if the bread box is full. I like eggs, too. Foolish me, I was nearly thirty years old before I resumed the habit of eating eggs for breakfast.

The complex and delicate egg is indispensable. Fried, scrambled, poached, or baked in a frittata, eggs make a meal on their own, and many wonderful dishes like mayonnaise and custard are impossible without them. But when the experts began to warn about cholesterol, the egg—specifically, the yolk—became a guilty pleasure; hence the culinary and nutritional abomination known as the egg white omelet. Eggs are rich in cholesterol, by the way, for the same reason breast milk is: cholesterol, among many other uses, is an essential part of cell membranes in mammals. That fact, however, was not enough to save the egg. In *Last Chance to Eat*, Gina Mallet writes of "the Egg Trauma."

> In the early 1970s, out of the blue, the American Heart Association declared the egg a threat to the heart. The egg contained 278 milligrams of cholesterol, and food scientists had just decreed that

> no one should consume more than 300 milligrams of cholesterol a day. The trauma that resulted lasted more than twenty years, almost crashed the egg industry, and turned what was then the largest egg-eating country in the world against eggs. The attack would prove to be a classic case of food science gone awry . . . I thought of course that the scientists, being scientists, had arrived at a safe level of dietary cholesterol through proof. How wrong I was.

Curious about the fate of the egg, Mallet interviewed Donald J. McNamara, a biochemist and the executive director of the Egg Nutrition Center, the egg industry lobby in Washington, D.C. She asked how scientists had arrived at the "safe" level of dietary cholesterol. "Dr. McNamara laughed," Mallet writes. "That was disconcerting." In 1968 food scientists met to sort out a safe amount of cholesterol to consume. Some were opposed to the very idea, while others firmly believed dietary cholesterol had a significant effect on blood cholesterol, and after much haggling they reached a compromise. The average intake of cholesterol was about 580 milligrams per liter of blood. Halving that, they settled on 300 milligrams—a political solution. "There's not one bit of scientific evaluation in that number," McNamara told Mallet.

We've known for some time that eggs are actually good for your heart. A study of 118,000 people reported in the *Journal of the American Medical Association* in 1999 was conclusive: "We found no evidence of an overall significant association between egg consumption" and heart disease. In fact, people who ate five or six eggs a week had a *lower* risk of heart disease than those who ate less than one egg per week.[1] The researchers, led by Walter Willet at the Harvard School of Public Health, cited a host of reasons fresh eggs might prevent heart disease: antioxidant carotenoids, vitamins, omega-3 fats, and good effects on blood sugar and insulin.

How did the egg get framed? Kudos to Gina Mallet for unearthing the origins of the arbitrary limit of 300 milligrams of cholesterol, which sparked three decades of unjustified fear. Our understanding of cholesterol is also more sophisticated now. We know that cholesterol metabolism—what the body *does* with LDL and HDL—is more important than the cholesterol in foods.

I was still curious about earlier studies apparently linking eggs and heart disease. Dr. Kilmer McCully, an expert on cholesterol metabolism, told me that real eggs weren't to blame. The studies used dehydrated eggs, which are liquidized, pasteurized, and spray-dried, in the same way powdered milk is made. Powdered eggs are mostly used in processed foods like cake mixes, but unfortunately the label won't say *powdered eggs.*

The cholesterol in powdered eggs (and powdered milk) is oxidized, which causes atherosclerosis. McCully says scientists have known since the 1950s that eating oxidized cholesterol causes atherosclerosis, but natural cholesterol does not.

The home cook who favors industrial convenience foods can buy powdered eggs, which last five or ten years. Here's the pitch from one company: "Our egg mix is mostly whole egg powder with a bit of powdered milk and vegetable oil . . . The egg mix has been formulated to make scrambled eggs, omelets or French toast. We think you'll find our egg mix a labor-saving food." No doubt, for some people, cracking open an egg is one chore too many, but I'm not sure you end up with more free time cooking with powdered eggs—just more omega-6 fats you don't need and lots of oxidized cholesterol.

Fresh eggs, by contrast, are a nutritional bonanza. Above all, eggs are a fine source of inexpensive protein. In fact, because the ratio of amino acids in eggs is so close to the ideal for human nutrition, eggs are the model for rating the quality of protein in all foods. Compared to meat and fish, eggs keep well. A fresh egg (ideally unwashed, with its protective film intact) will keep for two months in the fridge without much change in flavor or nutrition. An older egg will, however, be much easier to peel. This information comes in handy if you like your deviled eggs to look perfect—or if you think the farmer is putting you on about when they were laid.

A key ingredient in the egg yolk is lecithin, most famous as the emulsifier that makes mayonnaise creamy. Found in every human cell, lecithin helps the body digest fat and cholesterol. Lecithin is the source of choline, a B vitamin–like agent vital to the fetal brain. Eggs contain many antioxidants, including glutathione, which helps other antioxidants fight cancer and prevents oxidation of LDL. Yolks are extremely rich in the antioxidant carotenes lutein and zeaxanthin, which are good for the eyes (they prevent macular degeneration) and show promise in fighting colon cancer, and the lutein in eggs is more easily absorbed than the lutein also found in spinach.[2]

Along with liver, egg yolks have the highest concentrations of biotin—a B vitamin essential for healthy hair, skin, and nerves—of any food. Biotin is vital for digestion of fat and protein. Vitaminlike betaine is also abundant in eggs and liver. Betaine reduces homocysteine, an amino acid that causes atherosclerosis. All this makes chopped liver—the traditional Jewish paste of liver (chicken or beef), eggs, and chicken fat—very nutritious. It's a pity that many modern recipes for chopped liver call for corn oil instead of old-fashioned chicken fat, which is far better for you.

Eggs from pastured birds are superior to those from hens raised indoors, whose yolks are literally pale imitations of those from hens on grass. Pastured yolks are a rich yellow from the beta-carotene in plants. They also contain more monounsaturated fat, vitamins A and E, folic acid, lutein, and beta-carotene than indoor eggs. Pastured eggs are dramatically richer in omega-3 fats, which prevent obesity, diabetes, heart disease, and depression. The ratio of omega-6 to omega-3 fats in pastured eggs is ideal (about 1:1), while an indoor egg has almost twenty times more omega-6 than omega-3 fats. The omega-3 fats come from grass as well as insects, grubs, and worms. Another source is purslane, a lemony weed loved by poultry and foraging cooks alike. Along with walnuts and flaxseed, succulent purslane is a rare plant source of the omega-3 fat ALA. Some egg farmers feed flaxseed to indoor chickens to increase omega-3 fats.

WHY GRASS IS BEST: EGGS

	Monounsaturated fat (mg per g of yolk)	*Omega-3 fat (mg per g of yolk)*	*Ratio of omega-6: omega-3**
Hens raised indoors	115	1.73	19.4:1
Hens raised on grass	142	17.60	1.3:1

* The ideal ratio is 1:1

Source: Artemis Simopoulos, "Omega-3 Fatty Acids in Health and Disease and in Growth and Development," *American Journal of Clinical Nutrition,* Vol. 54 (1991): p.445.

Some eggs are advertised as "vegetarian." That may sound good, but it's actually not ideal. Recall that chickens are not natural vegetarians. Omnivores like us, they need complete protein and thrive on a diet of grain plus plenty of insects, worms, grubs, and other foods like sour milk. "Vegetarian" means the chickens were *not* fed cheap protein in the form of ground-up pigs, cattle, and poultry; that's good. But it also means something else. You may be certain that a vegetarian chicken has never been outdoors. If it had, it might have eaten a bug or two. If you can't find pastured eggs, barn-raised birds (not in cages) fed omega-3 are second-best.

The lesson of the egg trauma is simple. Don't eat factory eggs, powdered eggs, liquid eggs, pasteurized eggs, egg substitutes, or any other kind of industrial egg product somebody invented in the laboratory. Do eat the real thing: fresh, whole eggs from happy hens eating bugs and grubs outside on fresh green grass.

Whole Grains and Real Bread

PEOPLE ARE BEWILDERED BY FATS, but that's nothing compared with the welter of myths, half-truths, fears, and health claims around carbohydrates. Let me try to cut through the confusion. There are three macronutrients: protein, fat, and carbohydrate. Fat and protein, as we've seen, are essential for life. But no carbohydrate is essential. The body uses carbohydrates for energy, not structure or function, and it is theoretically possible to get all the energy you need from fat and protein. If calories aren't required, a highly sensitive hormone called insulin ensures that surplus carbohydrate is stored (with impressive efficiency) as fat—a little security against starvation in lean times. Because they don't cause insulin to rise quickly, fat and protein are less likely to be stored. This is the gist of low-carbohydrate diets.

None of this means that carbohydrates per se are bad for you. Let's talk about weight first. I'm afraid my advice is not original: eat as much carbohydrate as your body needs. How much that is depends on many things, including exercise and individual metabolism. My mother used to say, "If you're out in the cold or you work hard at physical labor all day, you can eat a lot of bread and rice." Some people gain weight easily on carbohydrates, while others can put away stacks of pancakes. A serving of pasta, rice, polenta, or oatmeal about the size of your fist is probably right for most people. It's crazy to count grams of carbohydrates in milk, carrots, or grapes. Even steak contains some carbohydrates. If you own a book listing those figures, throw it away. That's a recipe for neurosis.

There are indeed "good" and "bad" carbohydrates. "Complex" carbohydrates in whole foods are good, and "simple" carbohydrates like sugar are not. Eating sugar depletes B vitamins, which leads to premenstrual symptoms and depression, and promotes *Candida albicans,* a systemic yeast infection. Sugar also causes bone loss and, of course, tooth decay—but not for the reason you might think. Sugar upsets the balance of calcium and phosphorus, which causes teeth to rot from the *inside* out. Remember what the dentist Weston Price found when he studied people eating traditional and industrial foods? Poor nutrition—not lack of toothpaste—led to bone deformities and rotten teeth. Last but not least, by raising blood sugar, triglycerides, and cholesterol, sugar leads to obesity, diabetes, and heart disease. Of all the industrial foods, sugar is the most villainous.

Complex carbohydrates such as whole wheat and brown rice naturally contain B vitamins, vitamin E, and fiber. But even these complex carbohydrates are often refined. White or "polished" rice and white flour have been stripped of vitamins and fiber. After they remove the best parts (the bran and germ), only the starch, or carbohydrate, remains. The food industry prefers white flour because whole grain flour doesn't keep well; once grain is milled, wheat germ oil becomes rancid. White flour is fortified with synthetic B vitamins, but the vitamins in whole foods are superior. By the way, the bran and vitamin E taken from whole grains are fed to nutritionally deficient animals on factory farms. Animals on grass get all the fiber and vitamin E they need.

WHAT'S IN A GRAIN?

A grain—the starchy seed head of a grass—has three parts. *Whole grain* means the food contains all three. White flour contains only the endosperm, or starch. Grainlike foods, such as buckwheat, are often grouped with grains. They, too, are best whole.

- *Bran.* The hard protective coat; contains fiber, vitamins, and minerals.
- *Endosperm.* A complex carbohydrate wrapped in protein; the source of energy for a new plant.
- *Germ.* A tiny seed, capable of sprouting into a new plant; contains fat, protein, and vitamins.

The digestion of carbohydrate requires B vitamins. That's why the two nutrients are often found together in nature: whole wheat, brown rice, and beets (a major source of sugar) all contain B vitamins. When you eat white flour, white rice, or sugar, the body uses up B vitamins merely in the process of digestion. Thus, over time, refined carbohydrates deplete the body of B vitamins.

We have seen how carbohydrates cause blood sugar and insulin to spike more than fat and protein. Complex carbohydrates cause blood sugar to rise less quickly than simple ones because they must first be broken down into simple carbohydrates called *monosaccharides*. The simple carbohydrates (*mono-* and *disaccharides* such as sugar and juice) are small and able to enter the bloodstream rapidly. The larger complex carbohydrates (*polysaccharides* such as whole wheat) must be dismantled first. That takes time, so blood sugar rises slowly.

The fiber in complex carbohydrates further delays the spike in blood sugar. Fiber explains why an apple, even though it contains a lot of the simple carbohydrate fructose, is healthier than a soft drink sweetened with fructose—or even pure apple juice. In the apple, fructose comes with plenty of fiber.

Let me repeat: uneven blood sugar makes you fat. But even for slim people, steady blood sugar is desirable. Peaks and valleys in blood sugar also lead to diabetes and make you moody and lightheaded. With carbohydrates, this is my rule of thumb: *avoid the ones that go straight to your head.*

A SIMPLE GUIDE TO COMPLEX CARBOHYDRATES

All carbohydrates consist of monosaccharides and end up as monosaccharides after digestion. Complex carbohydrates may contain hundreds of monosaccharides, and they cause blood sugar to rise more slowly than simple ones. Fat and protein are even better for steady blood sugar.

Monosaccharides	*Disaccharides*	*Polysaccharides*
One saccharide	Two saccharides	Many saccharides
Simple	Simple	Complex
Very small	Small	Large
Enter blood instantly	Enter blood almost instantly	Enter blood slowly
Glucose	Sucrose and lactose	Cellulose and amylose
Sugar and fruit	Sugar and milk	Kale, carrots, and brown rice

The fiber, B vitamins, vitamin E, and antioxidants in whole wheat, brown rice, and other whole grains prevent obesity, diabetes, heart disease, and colon cancer. The government recommends three servings of whole grains daily, but the average American eats only one. The recent emphasis on the benefits of whole grains has led to an explosion of commercial whole grain breads, pasta, and baking mixes; quality is improving, too. For busy people and nonbakers, this is good news. The Oldways Preservation Trust, a food think tank, has devised the Whole Grains Stamp to alert buyers to foods containing whole grains.

Whole grain flour is nutritionally superior, but in certain baked goods, white flour gives a better texture. With pie crust, for example, you can just about get away with using one third whole wheat flour; add any more and the crust crumbles at the touch. You will have to make up your own mind about baked goods. For me, the occasional white flour crust (with lard and butter, of course) strikes an acceptable compromise between health and pleasure.

The complex carbohydrates in whole grains and legumes can be difficult to digest, causing bloating or cramps. Gluten intolerance, or celiac disease, is another problem common with wheat. All grains and legumes contain phytic acid, called an *antinutrient* because it reduces absorption of calcium, iron, magnesium, zinc, and other minerals. Other antinutrients in grains and beans, called *protease inhibitors*, interfere with protein digestion by blocking protease enzymes that break it down.

Yet these nutritional drawbacks have not stopped us from eating grains and beans. To aid digestion, reduce phytic acid, and increase nutrients, people all over the world sprout, soak, ferment, and cook corn, rice, wheat, and beans. All over the world, grains are a staple food for the poor. Dependence on grains would be catastrophic without these time-honored methods. In effect, foods are partially predigested by such kitchen tricks.

In the Americas, for example, conquistadores and colonists saw that the Aztecs soaked or ground corn with lime, but they didn't know why. Later, corn traveled to Europe without the tip about using lime, and people suffered for it. "Peasants who lived on corn throughout the winter came down with 'corn sickness,'" writes Betty Fussell in *The Story of Corn*. In 1771 an Italian named it *pellagra* (rough skin), but its cause remained mysterious. It was thought, perhaps, to be triggered by a kind of corn rot. Not until 1915, when the National Institutes of Health appointed Dr. Joseph Goldberger to investigate an epidemic of pellagra in the American South, did anyone suspect that pellagra was diet-related. Today we know that treating corn with lime (or some other alkali) liberates its vitamin B_3, and that pellagra is caused by lack of vitamin B_3, which is vital for metabolism.

Ancient cooks knew all this. An early recipe for cereals was pounded gruel. The Greeks ate a fermented, slightly alcoholic barley porridge, while Native Americans made a corn mush. After rudimentary porridge, the next development in grain cookery was unleavened bread. In the Old Testament, Ezekiel commands, "Take wheat, barley, beans, lentils, millet, and spelt and put them in one vessel and make bread of them." This passage also calls for sprouting the grains. Essene bread, a thin wafer of sprouted wheat flour, was probably the unleavened bread the Jews carried as they fled Egypt. Rich in vitamin C and protein, sprouts are remarkably nutritious, and many people who cannot digest wheat can eat sprouted grain breads, which are sold in whole foods shops.

Following traditional culinary and nutritional advice, I first soak the ground corn overnight with a pinch of baking soda when I'm making polenta, grits, or corn bread. According to Anson Mills, the miller of heritage varieties of American wheat, rice, and corn in Charleston, South Carolina, where I buy corn, lime also accentuates the floral flavors and aroma of grits. I soak rice for an hour and dried beans overnight, again with a pinch of soda. In effect, soaking is a mild form of fermentation.

THE OTHER WHOLE GRAINS

As with apples, pork, and every other food, monoculture reigns in grains. Today the dominant crops are wheat, corn, and rice, but this is a historical blip. For millennia, people have eaten dozens of others.

- *Amaranth.* An Aztec staple, amaranth has no gluten.
- *Barley.* Grown by the Egyptians, barley has a lot of fiber and needs long cooking. Pearled barley is slightly refined and cooks more quickly.
- *Buckwheat.* A cousin of rhubarb, not a grain, buckwheat contains the antioxidant rutin and is famous in American pancakes, Japanese soba noodles, and Russian kasha.
- *Kamut.* An ancient wheat with large, yellow, sweet grains. More protein and fats than durum wheat.
- *Millet.* A small, round grain with a delicate, nutty flavor, millet is a staple in India and delicious with butter.
- *Oats.* Buy whole rolled or steel-cut oats and soak overnight in water with a spoonful of yogurt or whey.
- *Quinoa.* Cultivated by the Incas, quinoa is a member of the beet family. Light and fluffy, it cooks quickly.
- *Rice.* One of the most easily digested grains, rice may be brown, red, or black.
- *Rye.* With more fiber than wheat, rye makes a dense bread and superior sourdough.
- *Spelt.* An ancient wheat, with more protein, it is often tolerated by people who can't eat wheat.
- *Teff.* A kind of millet with a very tiny, somewhat sweet grain, it is a staple in Eritrea and Ethiopia, where they make a spongy fermented pancake called *injera*.
- *Wild rice.* A swamp grass, not technically a rice, with a strong flavor and more fiber than rice.

The next development in grain cookery also used fermented grains, this time in the form of sourdough and yeast bread. The first leavened bread was invented by the Egyptians around 2300 BC. The early bakers let flour and water sit uncovered for several days, allowing it to bubble and expand from wild yeast spores in the air. Essentially, this is the same sourdough starter traditional bakers use today. Next, one adds flour and water to the starter, kneads the dough, and lets it rise with the action of the yeast. A good baker keeps a bit of starter for the next batch. Some starters have lasted for generations in the kitchen.

Natural, spontaneous leavening was the basic method of Western bread baking until the twentieth century, when commercial yeast was introduced. In 1961, bread suddenly became industrial with the invention of a technique by the Flour Milling and Baking Research Association in Chorleywood, England. The "Chorleywood bread process," as it is known, uses chemical improvers and low protein wheat, even though high protein wheat makes superior bread. Fermentation is dispensed with altogether. Unfortunately, "it's the fermentation time that makes bread digestible," says John Lister, a traditional miller at Shipton Mills, in the Cotswolds in England.[3] Real bread also tastes better.

Perhaps you think soaking corn meal in soda, or finding a bakery that makes proper bread, is quaint, peculiar, or just too much trouble. I hope not. It's worth the effort, for health and flavor. But my commitment to old foodways, as historians like to call these culinary legacies, is nothing compared to advocates of the Stone Age diet, whose view of the ideal diet is far more radical. They believe that bread itself—not only industrial bread—is bad for you, and it's worth hearing what they have to say.

In 1985, Dr. Boyd Eaton wrote a seminal article in the *New England Journal of Medicine* called "Paleolithic Nutrition." Eaton noted that high blood pressure, diabetes, heart disease, and cancer were rare among modern carnivorous hunter-gatherers such as the !Kung in the Kalahari Desert, aborigines in

Australia, and Ache in Paraguay. Loren Cordain, a professor at Colorado State University, was inspired by Eaton's work and decided that we should eat like Stone Age people. What does that mean?

In *The Paleo Diet*, Cordain calls for liberal amounts of green vegetables, fruit, fish, game, and pastured meat, poultry, and eggs. On that much, experts agree, but Cordain goes farther—right back to the Stone Age. His diet forbids all farmed foods, including grains, legumes, dairy, potatoes, and honey. Cordain is particularly critical of cereals, which he calls "nutritional lightweights" compared with meat, fish, and produce. Per calorie, meat and fish contain four times more vitamin B_3 than whole grains. A one-thousand-calorie serving of vegetables contains more calcium, magnesium, potassium, and iron than a similar serving of whole grain cereal. The vegetables also have five times more vitamin B_6, six times more B_2, and nineteen times more folic acid than whole grains.

When I delved into Stone Age nutrition, I was surprised to learn that the rise of farming was not entirely good news for human health. Archaeologists agree that early farmers had diseases and conditions not seen in hunter-gatherers, including parasites, syphilis, leprosy, tuberculosis, anemia, bone infections, and rickets. On the Neolithic diet, humans got shorter, a reliable sign of poor nutrition. Farming did cause a population boom—largely because grain is an inexpensive, easily stored source of calories—but general health declined.[4]

The proponents of Paleolithic diets have a point: the body does not require wheat, corn, chickpeas, or milk, which are relatively recent additions to the diet. All the essential nutrients are found in Stone Age foods. Given the emphasis on the nutritional value of whole grains today, it is perhaps surprising that you can get plenty of vitamins, minerals, and fiber without grains, but true. As for dairy, East Asian cultures thrive without it. Dr. Ben Balzer, an expert on Paleolithic nutrition, says that for the same calories, the typical hunter-gatherer diet has more vitamins, minerals, omega-3 fats, and antioxidants than the modern diet.

Americans do eat too many grains and refined grains. The main villain is corn, in three forms: corn-fed beef, corn oil, and corn syrup. On factory farms, cattle eat corn that is too rich in omega-6 fats; then we eat the beef and milk lacking the omega-3 fats we need. Corn oil, the main source of excess omega-6 fats, is a major cause of obesity, diabetes, and heart disease. Corn also becomes high fructose corn syrup, the main caloric sweetener in junk food. Intake of high fructose corn syrup grew by more than 1,000 percent between 1970 and 1990, far exceeding changes in consumption of any other food. The rise of corn syrup mirrors the increase in obesity.[5] Fructose also raises insulin, blood pressure, and triglycerides. If you take only one piece of advice from the Stone Age diet, stop eating all forms of industrial corn. It's far better to eat this delicious native vegetable in the traditional way: boiled with butter or in whole corn grits—ideally soaked first.

The Stone Age diet of whole foods has much to recommend it, but I'm not convinced it's necessary to give up all farmed foods. Our saliva and digestive tract contain enzymes such as amylase to digest starch. During the last Ice Age in North America, Siberia, and northern Europe, a wild wetland tuber called wapato was prolific, suggesting that ancient humans ate potatoes. What matters most is how we farm and how we prepare foods.[6]

I eat mostly Stone Age foods, but in my kitchen you'll also find traditional farmed foods, including sweet potatoes, raw milk cheese, lentils, whole grits, raw honey, and miso, a Japanese fermented soybean paste. I know we've been eating some of these foods for "only" two or four or ten or thirty thousand years—not three million—but that's long enough for me.

Traditional and Industrial Soy Are Different

IN MY VEGAN AND low-fat days, I was sometimes wistful for chocolate pudding, peach milk shakes, and apple pie à la mode. To satisfy my hankering for dairy, I bought soy "milk" and "ice cream." Millions of people began to eat soy foods, too—perhaps for the same reason. In supermarkets today, the soy milk section is almost as big as the dairy department, and that's no accident. Once soy milk appeared in the chilled dairy case, next to the milk, sales took off. Not long ago, the soy beverage was an odd creature, a canned drink for people on funny diets. Now, dressed in gable-top milk cartons, soy beverages look much like another kind of milk.

Long popular with vegetarians as a meat substitute, soy foods went mainstream with the rise of the "heart-healthy" diet. The U.S. government says twenty-five grams of soy protein daily, as part of a diet low in saturated fat and cholesterol, may reduce the risk of heart disease. Soy isoflavones are antioxidants, and its amino acids keep insulin in check. Soy may also prevent osteoporosis, hot flashes, prostate cancer, and some breast cancers.

These health benefits are impressive, and I began to wonder if the soy foods I was eating were traditional foods by my rough definition. Do they have a long history in the diet? Are they made pretty much the way they used to be? It turns out that some soy foods are traditional, others less so. This is what I learned about the remarkable soybean.

In China five thousand years ago, the soybean was grown to feed animals and build soil fertility, but not for human consumption. It turns out that we don't digest soybeans easily. In the Chou Dynasty (1134–246 BC), the Chinese learned to ferment soybeans to make them digestible to humans, and after this discovery, various fermented foods like Japanese miso sprang up. Bean curd was fermented, as in Chinese *sufu*, Indonesian tempeh, and Japanese *tofuyo*, or "spoiled milk."

Like all legumes, soybeans contain phytic acid, which, as we've seen, is called an antinutrient because it reduces absorption of calcium, iron, magnesium, zinc, and other minerals.[7] Diets high in phytic acid stunt growth. Cooking reduces phytic acid somewhat, and both soy milk and tofu are cooked. But fermentation is better; fermented tofu contains more available iron.[8] Soy also contains protease inhibitors, which interfere with protein digestion by blocking protease enzymes that break it down. Protease inhibitors are reduced by cooking or fermentation.[9]

At first the chemistry of soybeans seemed arcane to me, but the effects are important. After World War II, the United States sent soybeans to hungry people in Japan, Korea, and Germany. When the Germans got headaches and stomach pain and lost weight, the Americans, guessing they were biologically different from Asians, stopped sending soy. Later, U.S. scientists discovered the necessity of fermenting soybeans—only to find that Asians knew the secret all along.

Many people think that soy provides complete protein, but that's not quite so. Soy does have all the essential amino acids, but only trace amounts of two: cysteine and methionine. The body cannot make methionine. It can make cysteine, but only from methionine. Only animal products contain high-quality protein, with the right amount and proportion of all the amino acids. Soy is also said to contain vitamin B_{12}, but that's misleading. The compound in soy that resembles B_{12} cannot be used by the body. True vitamin B_{12} is found only in animal foods, with one partial exception. Some B_{12} is created during fermentation by microorganisms—which are, of course, tiny animals. Thus yeast and beer contain trace amounts of B_{12}. Vitamin B_{12} is essential, but a small quantity is enough. Eating fermented soy sauce may be one reason Asians were able to survive protein-poor diets during famines.

In the United States, the soybean was little known until the 1920s, when the government paid farmers to grow it. Animals on factory farms eat a lot of soybean cakes, but as a raw commodity, soybeans don't fetch a very high price. With a bit of tinkering, however, the soybean can be made much more profitable. In a remarkably short time, the food industry transformed the soybean from animal fodder into thousands of convenience foods worth billions of dollars.

The modern soybean yields two products for human consumption: oil and protein. Rare a hundred years ago, soybean oil is now the most popular oil in the world. In culinary-historical terms, it's an overnight sensation. Annually, Americans consume eighteen billion pounds of soybean oil, some 75 percent of the oil they eat. Alas, most soybean oil is industrial. About 85 percent of the U.S. crop is genetically engineered, and most of it is treated with heavy doses of nitrogen fertilizer and pesticides. Soybean oil is pressed under great heat and pressure, and the pulp is treated with solvents like hexane to extract the last drops of oil. The oil may be washed in lye, deodorized, and bleached. It's no surprise that industrial soybean oil emerges oxidized and carcinogenic.[10]

Cold-pressed oil from organic soybeans is better; its polyunsaturated fats and vitamin E are undamaged. However, soybean oil is rich (53 percent) in the omega-6 fat linoleic acid (LA), and as we've seen, we already eat too much LA. That's why soybean oil is the only soy food that Barry Sears, author of *The Soy Zone,* does *not* recommend. The flavor is nothing special, either, and olive oil contains all the omega-6 fats you need.

Unusually for a bean, the soybean contains more protein (38 percent) than carbohydrate. When soybean oil is made, a great deal of protein remains. Ingeniously, soy producers have transformed this leftover into the key ingredient in imitation sausages, milk, and cheese. Called soy protein isolate, it's 90 percent protein. As usual, industrial production does it no favors. Vitamins and the amino acid lysine are lost, while aluminum residue remains. Soy protein isolate does not have the FDA status known as GRAS (Generally Recognized as Safe).

With the invention of soy protein isolate, the market for soy foods exploded, and now it's the base for chips, pasta, meatless sausage, and dairylike foods. The challenge is making these imitation foods taste like the real thing. As fans of the tofu stir-fry know, the naturally bland soybean is a good platform for other flavors. It can also be "beany" or bitter. Texture is another problem: soy "cheese" is distinctly rubbery. Aware of all this, industry scientists are hard at work on soybean hybrids and processing methods to improve soy texture and flavor. Meanwhile, industrial soy foods need a boost in the flavor department. Typical ingredients in soy "ice cream" are sugar, corn oil, soy protein isolate, food starch, and flavoring. Fake cheese often contains hydrogenated oils, and MSG is common in savory foods like hot dogs.

Because flavor is not its strong suit, much of the soybean's appeal rests on health claims. Evidence for some benefits of soy seems strong. Soy isoflavones reduce LDL. As part of a diet low in refined carbohydrates, lean soy protein regulates blood sugar and insulin. That's the message of *The Soy Zone*, by Sears, who devised a soy diet (with, I noted, added fish oil and vitamin B_{12}) for his vegetarian daughter.

Asians have lower rates of osteoporosis than Americans, and some studies show higher bone density with soy-rich diets. Is soy responsible? It's not clear. Phytic acid in unfermented soy reduces calcium absorption.[11] In Asia and elsewhere, traditional diets also include calcium-rich bone broth and ample vitamin D, which is vital for calcium absorption. In fact, milk is far superior to soy as a source of calcium. One cup of soy drink has 10 milligrams of calcium, while milk has 300 milligrams, and more of the calcium in milk is absorbed.

Because soy is rich in isoflavones (plant estrogens), it's a natural remedy for symptoms of menopause. But the research is mixed.[12] Several recent studies have found that soy isoflavones were no better than a placebo in treating hot flashes. Moreover, large doses are not without risk; eating 60 grams of soy protein daily for only one month disrupts menstrual cycles.[13]

On soy and breast cancer, the data are voluminous, the claims competing, and the results unclear.[14] Some researchers believe soy *prevents* breast and prostate cancer, while others suggest it *causes* both. Genistein, the main soy isoflavone, can encourage cancer in breast cells, but genistein supplements are not necessarily equivalent to the genistein in whole soy foods.[15] In 2001, researchers who reviewed studies on soy and breast cancer said, "The honest response to each of these diametrically opposed claims is that no convincing data exist to support either claim."[16] It may be that the estrogens in soy are bad for estrogen-dependent breast cancer, but not other types of breast cancer.

Given the uncertainty, most experts recommend soy foods rather than isoflavone pills.[17] Foods may be superior because pills don't contain all the biological compounds originally in soy, but no one knows. The breast cancer specialist Dr. Susan Love, who believes soy can be beneficial, says that "soy food and soy supplements are not the same. Soy as food is probably safe for women with breast cancer, but the final answers aren't in yet."[18]

Soy should be viewed as part of a diverse diet, not as a nutritional silver bullet. The island of Okinawa, about four hundred miles off Japan, makes a fascinating case study for diet and disease. More Okinawans reach the age of one hundred than any other population in the world. Islanders have less heart disease, stroke, and cancer than mainland Japanese. Fans of soy note that Okinawans eat more soy protein than any other group: one hundred grams daily, versus forty grams on mainland Japan, and a mere four grams in the United States.

If food does account for the Okinawans' extraordinary health (which seems likely), I'm inclined to credit the *entire* diet—including raw fish, antioxidant tea, and traditional soy foods. Islanders also eat fewer calories, twice as much fish, and twice as many vegetables as mainland Japanese. An American wishing for the longevity of an Okinawan would need to do more than sprinkle one hundred grams of soy protein on his cereal. It's always better to eat real foods than pop pills. Soy protein reduces cholesterol, for example, but isoflavone supplements don't. An Okinawan proverb sums it up nicely: "One who eats whole food will be strong and healthy."[19]

In traditional Asian cuisine, soy is part of a diverse diet. Tofu is typically eaten with an animal protein such as fish broth, which provides complete protein and reduces the effects of phytic acid.[20] Many foods, such as natto, miso, and often tofu, are fermented. There is a bewildering variety of traditional tofu recipes. Indonesian tempeh, a chewy soy cake made with rice or millet, is quite unlike silky Japanese tofu, for example. In China, various pungent fermented tofus, pickled and aged in rice wine, chillies, and spices, are used in specific dishes, such as steamed pork and congee (a rice gruel).

The most famous fermented soy food is soy sauce. Traditionally, whole soybeans are slowly fermented to break down the protein and develop a distinctive briny flavor. Industrial soy sauce is made with defatted soy protein, wheat, sugar, preservatives, and coloring. Using defatted soybeans speeds fermentation because complex oils need not be broken down into fatty acids, but soy sauce made from defatted soy lacks the flavor, aroma, and health benefits of the real thing.

Edamame, an ancient Japanese delicacy of fresh, young, whole soybeans, is not a fermented soy food. The beans are merely boiled. Perhaps young beans are easier to digest than mature, dried beans and thus don't require fermentation; I don't know. Bright green *edamame* tastes a bit like a sweet young lima bean and is delicious with salt.

TRADITIONAL SOY FOODS

Many soy foods are common in more than one Asian country. For example, fermented bean sauce is originally Chinese, but it turns up in Vietnamese and Thai dishes. You will find the following foods in whole food shops, good grocers, and Asian markets.

- *Amazake*. Sweet, cultured rice "pudding" (Japanese).
- *Bean sauce*. Salty, fermented soybean sauce, often spicy.
- *Miso*. Salty, fermented paste of cooked soybeans, aged for a year or more (Japanese).
- *Natto*. Salty topping of fermented, cooked whole soybeans (Japanese).
- *Soy milk*. Soybeans are soaked, ground, simmered, and pressed.
- *Soy sauce*. Salty, aged, fermented condiment, best made with whole soybeans.
- *Sufu*. Fermented tofu condiment regarded as medicinal (Chinese).
- *Tahuri*. Fermented tofu (Filipino).
- *Tamari*. Liquid left after miso is made, used like soy sauce; contains no wheat (Japanese).
- *Tempeh*. Fermented tofu cake often containing rice or millet (Indonesia).
- *Tofu*. The traditional soybean curd; may be firm or soft, grainy or silky; often fermented.

- *Tofuyo.* Fermented tofu said to be good for the stomach (Japanese).

HEALTH BENEFITS OF FERMENTED SOY

- More digestible
- Less phytic acid (thus more minerals)
- Fewer protease inhibitors (thus more available protein)
- True vitamin B_{12}
- More isoflavones[21]

How much soy is beneficial? No one knows—or, rather, the experts don't agree. They can't even settle on how much soy was traditionally eaten in Asia or is eaten today. Proponents say daily consumption in Asia ranges from 40 to 100 grams of soy protein, but skeptics counter that Japanese and Chinese eat only 10 grams. Even allowing for differences in actual consumption within and between Asian countries, this wide range is probably due to selective reporting from the pro- or antisoy camps or both.

Fermentation is another factor. Critics argue that most soy in traditional diets was fermented, and for centuries it probably was, but unfermented soy is more common now. If fermented soy is better, any health benefits Asians enjoy may disappear as they begin to eat more industrial soy. Unfortunately, the following figures for actual, recommended, and maximum safe consumption don't distinguish between traditional and industrial soy. The best I can say for these wildly different numbers is this: they present an accurate—if frustrating—picture of the conflicting views about soy.

HOW MUCH SOY PROTEIN PER DAY? HARD TO SAY

	Grams Per Day
Estimate of the typical American diet	4
Estimate (by soy critic) of Japanese and Chinese diets	10

Recommended (*The Simple Soybean and Your Health*)	15
FDA-approved claim to help prevent heart disease	25
Thyroid suppression in healthy people	30
Upper limit for women (*The Simple Soybean and Your Health*)	30
Pre–breast cancer changes after fourteen days	38
Estimate (by soy proponent) of mainland Japanese diet	40
Recommended for vegetarian women (*The Soy Zone*)	40
Recommended for vegetarian men (*The Soy Zone*)	50
Menstrual disruption after one month	60
Upper limit for women (*The Soy Zone*)	75
Upper limit for men (*The Soy Zone*)	100
Estimate of Okinawa diet	100

HOW MUCH SOY PROTEIN IS IN A SERVING?

The following foods have about 30 grams of protein and just under 30 milligrams of isoflavones.

8 oz extra-firm tofu

12 oz firm tofu

16 oz soft tofu

4 oz soy "cheese"

24 oz soy "milk"

32 oz soy "yogurt"

30 g soy protein powder

Upper limits for safe consumption are important, because it is possible to eat too much soy. Excess genistein is toxic to the thyroid, which regulates appetite, metabolism, mood, and libido. In 1999, as the FDA was considering the claim that soy can prevent heart disease, two FDA specialists told the agency their concerns about hypothyroidism. They wrote, "There is abundant evidence that some of the isoflavones found in soy . . . demonstrate toxicity in estrogen-sensitive tissues and in the thyroid. Our conclusions are that no dose is without risk."[22] Japanese researchers found that 30 grams of roasted, pickled soybeans daily suppressed thyroid function in healthy people.[23] They called the dose "excessive." Yet proponents recommend 40 to 50 grams of soy protein daily.

One group is particularly vulnerable to soy: babies. Many studies confirm that soy causes hypothyroidism and goiter in babies. Soy formula may stunt growth and disrupt hormones, sexual development, and immunity. The dose of isoflavones in soy-based formula is huge: one thousand times greater than in breast milk.[24] New Zealand, Canada, Ireland, Switzerland, and Britain advise caution in feeding soy to babies. One of the FDA soy experts cited above called soy formula "a large, uncontrolled, and basically unmonitored human infant experiment."[25]

Soy is a complex food, and there are no easy answers. I certainly would not feed soy to babies or children, and would advise caution for adolescents, whose sexual development is incomplete. Vegetarians might consider what kind of soy foods they eat and how much, and women with breast cancer should consult a specialist familiar with the latest research. For me, industrial soy "milk" and other imitation foods flunk the real food test. This unique vegetable is more digestible, nutritious, and tasty when prepared in the traditional way. If you appreciate soy, do as Asian cultures have for two thousand years: eat traditional soy foods.

I Explain the Difference Between Good Salt and Bad

FOR THOUSANDS OF YEARS, salt has been central to human life. Greek slave traders traded salt for slaves, giving us the expression "not worth his salt," and Roman legionnaires were paid in salt; *salarium* is the Latin root of *salary*. In Sanskrit, *lavanya*, suggesting grace, beauty, and charm, comes from *lavana* for salt. Many wars have been fought over salt supplies, and many political battles over salt taxes. Like fish, salt was prized by landlocked people, who burned salty marsh grass and added the ash to food.

We seek salt for good reasons. Salt stimulates the gastric juices, and it's necessary to emulsify, or digest, fats. Hydrochloric acid in the stomach (for digesting meat) is made with salt. Unrefined salt contains the electrolytes sodium, potassium, and chloride, which are essential for every cell function, including blood pressure, nerve signals, and muscle action. Chronic salt deprivation causes weight loss, inertia, nausea, and muscle cramps. In the kitchen, meanwhile, salt is indispensable. It enhances flavor, even making sweet things sweeter. Salt is a preservative, aids fermentation, and improves the texture of bread and cured meat.

Today, however, salt has a bad reputation. The psychology professor Paul Rozin has found that many Americans regard salt (and fat) as a toxin and believe even a trace amount is unhealthy. "This belief establishes a goal that is both extremely unhealthy, and unattainable," he says. Early studies *did* correlate salt intake and high blood pressure, but more recent research has been kinder to salt. In 1983, studies in the United States and Japan found that dietary salt didn't affect blood pressure in most people significantly.[26] In the 1990s, several U.S. and British studies concluded that salt itself is not the cause of poor health.[27]

In 2006, data from the prestigious NHANES II study showed that death from heart disease and from all causes *rose* with lower sodium consumption.[28] "Evidence linking sodium intake to mortality outcomes is scant and inconsistent," said the researchers. Yet doctors still routinely prescribe low-sodium diets for patients with hypertension and heart disease. According to Dr. Kilmer McCully, only a few people—about 20 percent—are "salt-sensitive." For most of us dietary sodium doesn't seem to affect blood pressure or heart disease risk. Meanwhile, many other factors raise blood pressure: too little potassium, stress, smoking, being overweight, and lack of exercise.

Three million years ago, Stone Age humans got all the salt they needed from eating meat and blood, fish, and sea vegetables; perhaps they occasionally dipped foods into seawater for salt. Later—probably around the time they began to eat more grain and other starches—humans became salt farmers, mining ancient seabeds for salt from the earth or gathering it from seawater. Archaeological evidence suggests that about four thousand years ago, humans produced salt in central China. Consumption of unrefined salt predates industrial diseases.

My friend Daniel Gevaert, who worked on our farm as a teenager many summers ago, taught me to appreciate real salt. Back home in France, he became an organic farmer, manufactured fermented soy foods, and bought a sea salt factory. *Factory* is not quite the right word, in that nothing much industrial happens there. From June to September, Atlantic sea salt is harvested manually with clay pans and allowed to dry naturally in the wind and sun. The factory is a simple shed, empty but for a chute. The salt dries gently as it flows along the chute, through screens that sort it into fine or coarse grains. The salt is never washed, heated, or refined in any way, and nothing is added.

A few years ago, Daniel and his wife, Valerie, sold Danival, the company they founded, to a large French concern. That made me a little sad, but it will be several years before I finish the salt from my last visit to the factory near Bordeaux. Daniel's salt is a soft gray and slightly moist. It is rich in minerals and trace elements, with an exquisite briny flavor. (Danival and other unrefined sea salts are sold in the United States under the brand Celtic.)

Typical commercial salt, by contrast, is an industrial leftover. First the chemical industry removes the valuable trace elements and heats it to twelve hundred degrees Fahrenheit. We get what's left: 100 percent sodium chloride, plus industrial additives, including aluminum, anticaking agents to keep the salt pouring smoothly, and dextrose, which stains it purple. Salt is then bleached. Consuming pure sodium chloride strains the body, upsetting fluid balance and dehydrating cells.

Unrefined sea salt is 82 to 84 percent sodium chloride, and the rest is other good stuff: calcium, magnesium (about 14 percent), and more than eighty trace elements including iodine, potassium, and selenium. These nutrients have vital functions, among them maintaining a healthy fluid balance and replenishing electrolytes lost in sweat. We need trace elements in tiny amounts, but a deficiency is serious. The landlocked American Midwest, for example, was known as the "goiter belt" for lack of iodine-rich seafoods. Today commercial salt contains added iodine to prevent thyroid disease, but the body absorbs natural iodine in unrefined salt more easily.

How much salt do you need? That depends on many things, including your size and genes and how much you sweat. As with fat (and carbohydrates and the rest), I don't count sodium milligrams, and I have no idea how much potassium a head of lettuce contains, but I know that eating a lot of fruits and vegetables is a good thing. I also know when I've eaten too much salt, just as sure as I know when I've put too much olive oil on the salad. The main clue? I'm thirsty.

The body needs a balance of the two main electrolytes, sodium and potassium. Whole foods contain little sodium and plenty of potassium, but the typical industrial diet is the opposite: it contains too much sodium and too little potassium. Do avoid sodium-rich industrial foods, including prepared meals, savory snacks, bouillon cubes, and commercial chicken stock. According to the National Academy of Sciences, processed food—not the salt cellar—accounts for 80 percent of the salt in the typical diet. When I do buy canned goods such as tomatoes and chickpeas, I look for unsalted versions, or I rinse the beans and add real salt to taste during cooking.

If you avoid industrial foods, exercise, eat fresh fruits and vegetables daily, and drink plenty of water, there is no need to fear traditional salt. In the kitchen and at the table, I'm liberal with unrefined salt. But remember: if you want the benefits of all the vital trace elements of the sea, the label should say *unrefined.* Salt sold simply as "sea salt" is refined in some way, no matter how charming and rustic the packaging. And yes, unrefined sea salt is more expensive than the rest. It's worth more.

Chocolate: The Darker the Better

EVERY WINTER, AROUND FEBRUARY 14, the food and health pages run amusing pieces on why women crave chocolate, or how it came to be associated with love and romance—and might even get you some. I used to find these reruns tedious, especially when they used the term *chocoholic,* but I have new respect for chocolate, which I consider one of the great food-drugs, along with wine and cayenne peppers. Now I skip the sexy quotes and scan the articles for hard facts on the dark, complex bean of the cacao tree, a native of lush jungles around the equator, from Hawaii to Venezuela to Nigeria. The tree and bean are called *cacao*—rhymes with *cow.* The liquor, powder, and drink are *cocoa.*

Everyone has his poison (or ought to), and I'd probably eat chocolate no matter what, but for chocolate lovers seeking nutritional validation, here is a sneak preview at the good news: the saturated and monounsaturated fats in cocoa butter are good for cholesterol; cocoa powder is rich in antioxidants and contains mild antidepressants.

Twelve hundred years before Christ, the Olmec of modern Mexico grew cacao trees and made the beans into a drink laced with chilies, herbs, and honey. The Mayans and Aztecs believed the God of Agriculture brought the cacao tree from paradise. At weddings, they served a cocoa drink called *xocalatl* (warm or bitter liquid), admired for its ability to enhance energy, passion, and sexual performance. In 1527, Hernán Cortés found the cocoa bean in Montezuma's court and took it home to Spain, where it was doctored with sugar and vanilla.

Soon chocolate spread pleasure across Europe, and in 1753 the Swedish naturalist Carolus Linnaeus renamed the cacao tree *Theobroma cacao*, Greek for "elixir of the gods." But chocolate lovers were not content to leave the divine bean alone; they wanted to perfect it. In 1879, chocolate was rendered smooth and creamy by conching, a trick devised by Rodolphe Lindt of Berne, Switzerland, one of many chocolate inventor-industrialists. A small producer in Sicily called Bonajuto sells the grainy, unconched kind made with the nineteenth-century method. It didn't knock me out when I tried it. I'm all for traditional methods of production, but to me, Lindt was a genius; with chocolate, I think, the smoother, the better.

HOW CACAO BEANS BECOME CHOCOLATE

First cacao beans are removed from the pods. The best chocolate makers ferment the beans to develop flavor. Next the beans are roasted (again for flavor), shelled, and broken up into little shards called nibs. Nibs are then ground and heated to make cocoa liquor. If you remove all the cocoa butter from the liquor, what's left is pure cocoa powder. If you add more cocoa butter, plus sugar and vanilla, to the liquor, you get a chocolate bar.

The cacao tree is an unusual plant. Cocoa powder contains large amounts of calcium, copper, magnesium, phosphorus, and potassium, and more iron than any vegetable. It is very rich in polyphenols, particularly a group called flavonoids, which account for the rich pigment in red wine, cherries, and tea. These antioxidants promote vascular health, prevent LDL oxidation, lower blood pressure, reduce blood clots, and fight cancer. A one-and-a-half-ounce (40-gram) bar of milk chocolate contains as many antioxidants as a five-ounce (150-ml) glass of red wine. Polyphenols are found in cocoa solids, not cocoa butter. Thus pure cocoa powder has the most antioxidants by weight, then dark chocolate, and finally milk chocolate. White chocolate—made of cocoa butter without any cocoa powder—has none at all.

The polyphenols in chocolate may prevent obesity, diabetes, and high blood pressure—all risk factors for heart disease. In 2005, the *American Journal of Clinical Nutrition* reported that eating three and a half ounces (100 grams) of dark chocolate daily decreased blood pressure and significantly improved sugar metabolism by increasing sensitivity to insulin. Insulin sensitivity is desirable; recall that in diabetes, the cells are deaf to insulin. White chocolate did not have the same effect.[29]

ANTIOXIDANTS IN CHOCOLATE AND OTHER FOODS

Each of the following contains about 200 milligrams of polyphenols. Note that chocolate from fermented beans contains more polyphenols, and dark chocolate contains more polyphenols than milk chocolate.

- 1.5 oz milk chocolate
- 1 glass red wine (5 oz)
- 12 glasses white wine (5 oz each)
- 2 cups tea
- 4 apples
- 5 servings of onions
- 3 glasses black currant juice
- 7 glasses of orange juice

Source: John Ashton and Suzy Ashton, *A Chocolate a Day Keeps the Doctor Away*.

The fats in chocolate—mostly monounsaturated and saturated—are also healthy. Chocolate is unctuous because cocoa butter melts at mouth temperature. The better chocolate bars have added cocoa butter, which is roughly equal parts stearic, palmitic, and oleic acid. Extra stearic acid is converted to oleic acid, so the net effect of these fats is good for cholesterol. A 2004 study in *Free Radical Biology and Medicine* found that chocolate increased HDL and reduced oxidation of cholesterol. Oxidized cholesterol causes atherosclerosis. Chocolate keeps well because saturated fats are stable, and any oxidation from heat or light is inhibited by cocoa's abundant polyphenols.

COCOA BUTTER IS GOOD FOR YOUR HEART

Oleic acid	***Stearic acid***	***Palmitic Acid***
Monounsaturated	Saturated	Saturated
Lowers LDL	Lowers LDL	Lowers cholesterol
Leaves HDL intact	Converts to oleic acid	Lowers LDL

Is chocolate addictive? The Chocolate Information Center—a research lab funded by the Mars company—prefers to call the craving for chocolate a "strong desire." "Theoretically," its scientists write cautiously, chocolate could "contribute to feelings of well-being." Chocolate contains the stimulants theobromine and caffeine; tyramine and phenylethylamine, which are uppers; and anandamide, which mimics cannabinoids, natural pain killers. (Anandamide derives from the Sanskrit *ananda*, "internal bliss.") But the chocolate scientists note that these natural drugs are found only in trace amounts in chocolate. Moreover, they are also found in many foods we don't crave. Caffeine is an exception; it is certainly habit-forming, but there is much more caffeine in coffee and tea than in chocolate.

Craving a certain food is sometimes regarded as signaling an acute nutritional deficiency, but in the case of chocolate, I'm not convinced. Chocolate is rich in magnesium. If a woman needs—and thus craves—magnesium before her period, she might just as easily have a strong desire to eat magnesium-rich foods, like broccoli, tofu, and kidney beans. Rushing to the corner shop for broccoli, however, is not part of PMS folklore.

What often goes unmentioned in discussion about the desire for chocolate is sugar. I suspect that sugar plays a large part in the urge to finish a bar of chocolate once you've torn into it. Sugar quickly brings on a gentle high, which is why so many people crave it in low moments. Unfortunately, the high is often followed by a crash.

Studies show that capsules containing the compounds in cocoa don't satisfy the desire as well as real chocolate, which strongly suggests that the aroma, flavor, and creaminess of chocolate, more than any mood-enhancing chemicals, are key factors in chocolate craving. In *Chocolate: A Bittersweet Saga of Dark and Light*, Mort Rosenblum considers all these factors, including the mood-enhancing agents in chocolate, and concludes that chocolate fails the two tests of addiction: "It is not dangerous to the human organism. And no symptoms of withdrawal appear when consistently high consumption is abruptly stopped."

NAKED CHOCOLATE

Nibs are little pieces of fermented, roasted, and shelled cacao beans—the raw material of all chocolate. More like nuts than candy, crunchy nibs are about half cocoa butter. They have a tannic flavor, like espresso or red wine. Try them in place of chocolate chips in cookies and brownies or sprinkle on ice cream. Toss nibs on roasted pumpkin or add to Mexican mole. They pack a little jolt of caffeine.

How much chocolate is good for you? John Ashton and Suzy Ashton, the authors of *A Chocolate a Day Keeps the Doctor Away*, who are unabashed enthusiasts, recommend no more than two ounces (55 grams) of chocolate each day, preferably dark chocolate, which has less sugar and more antioxidants. It also has more flavor than milk chocolate, which is why connoisseurs the world over prefer it. Once you're used to the bold, complex flavors of chocolate unmasked by sugar, the average milk chocolate will seem cloying. Not, I hasten to add, that there is anything wrong with milk, which goes very nicely with chocolate. After all, ganache is nothing more than blended cream and chocolate. If you like milk chocolate, look for a bar with more cocoa than sugar, such as one made by Scharffen Berger, which is 41 percent cocoa, about twice the amount in a typical bar.

Sugar makes me fat and grumpy, so gradually I weaned myself from dark (70 percent cocoa) to very dark (85 percent) chocolate bars. Occasionally, I will make a cup of cocoa with unsweetened chocolate and very fresh grass-fed raw cream, which is just sweet enough to balance the bitterness. Do buy the best unsweetened and dark chocolate you can afford; without sugar there is no concealing shoddy chocolate. Cheap chocolate can be bitter or metallic.

With chocolate desserts I recommend the same thing: less sugar. When you make chocolate mousse (or any dessert), use half the sugar called for. You will taste the chocolate first, instead of the sugar. When sweetness is not the dominant sensation, your appreciation for a particular flavor will grow; chocolate may seem fruity, smoky, or herbal, for example. Other flavors will change subtly, too. Next to dark chocolate, savory foods such as almonds, coconut, and cream are almost sweet. If you're used to sugary desserts, you may find "half-the-sugar" desserts not quite to your taste at first. But I swear by this rule of thumb. I follow it every time I try a new recipe for ice cream or pumpkin pie or anything else. As my mother likes to say, "If it's sweet on the first bite, it will be too sweet by the last."

9

Beyond Cholesterol

What Is Cholesterol?

WHEN I TOLD MY FRIEND Wendell Steavenson, an Anglo-American writer, I was writing a book about why butter is good for you, her comment was typically arch. "Cholesterol," she said, mock solemn, "only *exists* in America." I knew exactly what she meant. In much of the world—perhaps Wendy was thinking of London, Baghdad, Beirut, or Tbilisi, to name but a few cities where she has lived—people aren't morbidly afraid of traditional foods like cream and lamb. Not yet, anyway.

The American anticholesterol campaign, which British experts gently mock as "know-your-number" medicine, baffles foreigners. Here at home, it mostly inspires anxiety. When you sit down to eat with health-conscious Americans, the subject of cholesterol is hard to avoid, but the conversation seldom moves beyond weak jokes about clogged arteries.

We have been taught to fear this scoundrel called cholesterol, and fear it we do, yet most people have no idea what cholesterol is. It is often called a fat, but cholesterol is actually a sterol, a kind of alcohol. Cholesterol is part of all animal cell membranes. It makes up much of brain and nervous tissue, and it's an important part of organs including the heart, liver, and kidney. It is so vital to the developing brain that defects in cholesterol metabolism cause mental retardation.[1] Cholesterol is necessary to make vitamin D, bile acids (which digest fats), adrenal hormones, and the sex hormones estrogen and testosterone.

These roles are well known, at least to cholesterol experts. Then, in a college textbook, I came across a striking statement: cholesterol is a *repair* molecule. At first I didn't understand it—or quite believe it. After all, cholesterol is known for doing damage, not healing. But apparently that's not quite how cholesterol works. Let me explain by introducing the famous lipoproteins.

Low-density lipoprotein (LDL), often called the "bad" cholesterol, and its counterpart, high-density lipoprotein (HDL), or "good" cholesterol, are not forms of cholesterol at all, but vehicles. Like little boats with a waxy cargo, LDL and HDL ferry cholesterol around the body. LDL carries cholesterol from the liver to the tissues (including blood), and HDL carries cholesterol from the tissues back to the liver.[2] In every healthy person, the lipoproteins help cholesterol go about its chores, digesting fats here and making estrogen there. The body needs both LDL and HDL. According to the *Journal of American Physicians and Surgeons*, the "good" and "bad" cholesterol story is "overly simplistic and not supported by the evidence."[3]

Repair is one of cholesterol's many tasks. When arterial walls are damaged, cholesterol rushes to the scene on a dinghy piloted by LDL to fix them.[4] As the authors of *Human Nutrition and Dietetics* describe low-density lipoproteins, "their role is to deliver cholesterol to tissues for the vital functions of membrane synthesis and repair." In *Know Your Fats*, Mary Enig writes: "Cholesterol is used by the body as a raw material for the healing process. This is the reason injured areas in the arteries (as in atherosclerosis) or the lungs (as in tuberculosis) have cholesterol along with several other components (such as calcium and collagen) in the 'scar' tissue [they've] formed to heal the 'wound.'"

This would explain why high LDL is sometimes linked to heart disease. Many people with heart disease have damaged arteries, and cholesterol travels on LDL to heal them. Just because you see fire fighters at burning buildings does not mean they start fires.

Cholesterol comes from two sources. The body makes cholesterol in the brain and the liver, which makes about 1,500 milligrams daily. The other source is the diet. Only animal foods contain cholesterol. It is stored in the fat of dairy foods and the muscle of animal protein. Thus beef, pork, and poultry, although they vary in fat content, have similar amounts of cholesterol (about 20 milligrams per ounce). That means trimming the fat from meat will reduce the fat but not cholesterol content, whereas skim milk contains less cholesterol than whole milk. Egg yolks and milk are particularly rich in cholesterol because baby animals need large amounts to build brain cells.

Experts once thought that eating cholesterol raised blood cholesterol. In 1968, they advised us to limit dietary cholesterol to 300 milligrams daily. This figure was not only unrealistic—with 275 to 300 milligrams of cholesterol, eating one egg would put you at or near the limit—but also arbitrary, as Gina Mallet discovered. Now we know that blood cholesterol is largely determined by metabolism—how the body makes, uses, and disposes of cholesterol. "The amount of cholesterol in food is not very strongly linked to cholesterol levels in the blood," says a report from the Harvard School of Public Health.[5]

How much cholesterol do you need to eat? In theory, none; your body will make enough. But there are good reasons to consume cholesterol, which is harmless in its natural form. First, infants and children under two don't produce enough; cholesterol *must* be part of their diets, which is why breast milk has plenty.[6] The second reason to consume cholesterol applies to all ages: avoiding it entirely would mean shunning highly nutritious foods. Liver, meat, shrimp, butter, and eggs offer complete protein, omega-3 fats, and vitamins A, B_{12}, and D—all vital nutrients not found in plants. It is not possible to separate the cholesterol from the nutrients in these foods. Older people may even benefit from eating cholesterol. In 1995, researchers found that cholesterol in eggs aids older people with declining memory.[7]

The body aims to keep cholesterol levels steady. Thus the more cholesterol you eat, the less the liver makes, and the less you eat, the more the liver makes. That explains why vegans and vegetarians, who eat few animal foods or none at all, can have high cholesterol. Moreover, up to 50 percent of cholesterol is determined by genes, not diet.[8] As people with a family history of high blood cholesterol know, diet has little effect on blood levels.

If you have normal cholesterol metabolism, you may eat real foods without fear. As we've seen, people who eat traditional foods rich in cholesterol and saturated fat don't have high cholesterol or more heart disease. Other traditional foods, meanwhile, have salutary effects on health in general and heart disease in particular; they include fish, red wine, chocolate, and olive oil.

Industrial foods are the real villain in heart disease. The main offenders are trans fats, corn oil, and sugar. As we've seen, trans fats promote atherosclerosis and clotting; polyunsaturated vegetable oils lower HDL; and sugar depletes B vitamins and raises triglycerides. All these effects are bad for the heart. The actual culprits are easy to spot for anyone who cares to read more than casually about diet and heart disease. So why did a perfectly useful molecule called cholesterol, which we've been consuming in liver, eggs, and shrimp for three million years, take the fall?

How Cholesterol Became the Villain

THE IDEA THAT DIET contributes to heart disease is not new. In 1908, a young Russian medical researcher, M. A. Ignatovsky, fed rabbits a diet of animal protein, and when the bunnies developed arteriosclerosis, he blamed the protein. In 1913, a group of rival doctors followed by feeding cholesterol to rabbits, with similar results, including fat and cholesterol deposits in arteries, and they guessed that cholesterol, not protein, was responsible for the arteriosclerosis in Ignatovsky's rabbits as well as theirs.

Animal experiments can, of course, be very useful, but in this case researchers may have reached the wrong conclusions. Unlike humans, who are born to eat cholesterol, rabbits are herbivores with no ability to metabolize it. When you force-feed rabbits with cholesterol, their blood cholesterol rises ten or twenty times higher than the highest values ever seen in humans; the effect is like poisoning. "Cholesterol is deposited in the arteries of the rabbit, but these deposits do not even remotely resemble those found in human atherosclerosis," says Dr. Uffe Ravnskov, the author of *The Cholesterol Myths*.

Later, in human trials, researchers *deliberately* used oxidized cholesterol to demonstrate that dietary cholesterol causes atherosclerosis. Oxidized cholesterol, like oxidized or rancid polyunsaturated vegetable oil, is damaged and unhealthy. As I've mentioned elsewhere, it's no secret in cholesterol circles that oxidized cholesterol, found in powdered eggs, powdered milk, and fried foods, causes arterial plaques.[9] Dr. Kilmer McCully, author of *The Heart Revolution,* says that "pure cholesterol, containing no oxy-cholesterols, does not damage arteries in animals."

Nevertheless, by the 1950s the cholesterol theory was well established: it was thought that eating cholesterol raises blood cholesterol and causes arteriosclerosis. Then, in a significant development, researchers concluded that cholesterol was not acting alone. The revised cholesterol theory had two parts: first, saturated fats (as opposed to unsaturated fats) raise cholesterol, and second, elevated cholesterol causes arteriosclerosis.

Ancel Keys, the professor we met in an earlier chapter on fats, led the campaign against saturated fats. A prolific writer and speaker, Keys spent his last years in Naples, presumably enjoying the Mediterranean diet he had become famous for promoting. When he died in 2004, at the age of one hundred, his influence on diet and disease was rightly considered vast. Theodore Van Itallie wrote this tribute in *Nutrition and Metabolism*: "For those of us who worked . . . to call attention to the relationship of serum total cholesterol to risk of coronary heart disease (CHD), and to the cholesterol-raising effects of certain saturated fats, Keys will always be one of the major prophets who provided the early evidence that atherosclerosis is not an inevitable concomitant of aging, and that a diet high in saturated fat . . . can be a major risk factor for CHD."[10]

In the 1950s, Keys made a series of contradictory statements about fats.[11] He said that all fats raise cholesterol; yet elsewhere, he wrote that saturated fats raise cholesterol and polyunsaturated oils lower it. Keys said that animal fats caused heart disease; elsewhere, he wrote there was no difference between animal fats and vegetable oils in their effects. Clearly, his data were inconsistent. Nevertheless, Keys focused on one hypothesis: that a diet high in fat and saturated fat caused heart disease.

In 1953, Keys published a famous paper known as the Six Countries Study, placing fat and cholesterol at the center of the debate about diet and heart disease. Keys presented a diagram of fat consumption and death from heart disease in six countries; it appeared to show that the more fat people ate, the more deaths from heart disease. Japan was at the low end of the graph, which swept smoothly upward, and the United States was at the top. But the diagram didn't tell the whole story. There were, in fact, data on fat and heart disease from twenty-two countries, but Keys omitted the other sixteen.[12] Instead of forming a convincing upward curve, the twenty-two data points were scattered all over. He declined to cite Finland and Mexico, for example, where fat consumption was similar. Finland had seven times the rate of heart disease as Mexico.

In 1970, Keys published another famous paper—the Seven Countries Study—which appeared to demonstrate a link between cholesterol and heart disease in fifteen populations in seven countries. "The correlation is obvious," said Keys. But when Ravnskov plotted Keys's raw data into a graph, the correlation fell apart. The link is even weaker when you compare groups within countries. On the Greek island of Corfu, for example, people died five times more often from a heart attack than their fellow Greeks living on nearby Crete, although cholesterol on Corfu was lower.

Keys was undeterred and went on to advocate what he called the Mediterranean diet. "The heart of what we now consider the Mediterranean diet is mainly vegetarian," he wrote. "Pasta in many forms, leaves sprinkled with olive oil, all kinds of vegetables in season, and often cheese, all finished off with fruit and frequently washed down with wine." But the traditional Mediterranean diet is not chiefly vegetarian; beef, lamb, goat, pork, game, poultry, liver, and fish are common fare.

Pork—to name only one meat—is eaten throughout the region, where pigs (never fussy eaters) thrive on scrubby land. Italy and Spain are famous for cured pork (prosciutto and serrano ham) and for sausages, which require extra lard. The Spanish make sweet lard cakes called *mantecados*, while Italian bakers use *strutto* (rendered lard) much the way American and British cooks once did. In Tuscany, *lardo di Colonnata*—lard aged in marble with herbs—is eaten straight. In France, warm pork fat dressing and some kind of bacon are de rigueur in the classic salads *pissenlit au lard* and *frisée aux lardons*, made with the bitter greens dandelion and endive, respectively.

Olive oil is also traditional in the Mediterranean, of course. It's eaten liberally on Crete, for example. ("My God, how much oil you use!" Keys is said to have exclaimed when he saw a green salad drowning in olive oil on the island.) But traditional Mediterranean cuisine includes many other fats, too. In northern Italy, butter is typical, and lard is eaten in central regions. In sprawling Provence, which spans the Mediterranean coast and the Alps, olive oil and lard are common, and Gascons are famous for duck and goose fat.

Although Keys was a central figure in the cholesterol hypothesis, he was not always invited to mingle with the nutrition establishment. Some people think this relative ostracism was due to his loner character and indifference to politics. I wonder whether Keys was excluded because proponents of the cholesterol hypothesis were threatened by his lifelong habit of independent thinking.

The medical professor Stephen Phinney remembers a hallway encounter with Keys in the mid-1980s, shortly after the Lipid Research Clinic Coronary Prevention Trial demonstrated that the drug cholestyramine reduced cholesterol and coronary mortality. Keys showed Phinney a paper in which he examined HDL and mortality in Minnesota businessmen. In the paper, Keys wrote that HDL levels predicted heart-related deaths, but not death from all causes. Phinney recalled: "Dr. Keys was fuming, because this manuscript had been rejected by the major medical journals. Having set the cholesterol-lowering juggernaut in motion, the nutrition establishment was not about to let him sully the picture by demonstrating that it was not the only factor that determined important outcomes such as longevity. In his early 80s, Dr. Keys was still way out ahead of the consensus."[13]

Later, Phinney told me why Keys, a nutritional epidemiologist, was unique in his field. "He understood the complexity of nutritional metabolism, whereas the pharmacologists either sought to reduce its complexity or ignored it. Pharmacology is a reductionist discipline—you always want to purify your drug and precisely define its target and its mechanism," said Phinney. "This helps explain why diet and nutrition struggle for acceptance in the medical mainstream. The Mediterranean diet works better than atorvastatin"—the statin sold as Lipitor, which lowers LDL—"because it breaks the reductionist rule by harnessing the power of a combination of nutrients working against both cholesterol and inflammation."[14]

Ancel Keys left a substantial legacy—and a complicated one. He was right to praise antioxidant-rich vegetables, monounsaturated olive oil, and fish. In 1994, the famous Lyon study found the greatest protection against heart disease in the Mediterranean diet was provided by omega-3 fats found in fish.

Yet Keys also set the stage for a battle against the alleged dangers of saturated fats in traditional foods such as butter—dangers that were oversold, if not by Keys himself then certainly by the medical-pharmaceutical complex, which took up the anticholesterol campaign with enthusiasm befitting a crusade.

The Cholesterol Skeptics

THE OLD ADVICE—butter ⇒ high cholesterol ⇒ heart attack—was too crude to be accurate. New advice is more subtle; even the conventional wisdom holds that margarine is "worse than" butter, and we know that high HDL is good. Yet I have some sympathy for the researchers who reduced the message to an antibutter slogan. They meant well. If you labor in a complex field—and heart disease is certainly that—the appetite for simple answers can be maddening.

People will ask, If butter doesn't cause heart disease, what does? Well, I venture, genes, lack of exercise, inflammation, free radicals, smoking, and industrial foods like trans fats, sugar, and corn oil. I believe this is accurate and reasonably complete; I hope it's also brief enough to keep people from nodding off. I don't envy doctors, who are forced by the clock and by anxious patients to reduce complex disease etiology, diagnosis, and treatment to three-minute summaries.

On diet and disease, this is as simple as I can make it without doing injustice to accuracy or uncertainty: *traditional foods are good for you*. There are various ways to go about proving this. You can feed people corn or coconut oil, and see that corn oil lowers HDL and coconut oil doesn't. You can observe whether people who eat extreme diets (e.g., all meat) get heart disease. And so on. Such studies convinced me that you can eat whatever you want—except industrial foods. If that satisfies you, close this book and enjoy butter and eggs. Those who would like to know more about heart disease may wish to read on.

The quintessential disease of civilization, heart disease was rare before 1900, and rare it remains in preindustrial groups. In the United States, the first heart attack was reported in 1912, and by midcentury heart disease was the nation's biggest killer. Today cardiovascular diseases—conditions of the heart and blood vessels, including angina, stroke, congestive heart failure, and heart disease—are still the leading cause of death. All cardiovascular diseases combined kill about a million Americans a year, men and women in pretty much equal numbers. Heart disease alone is responsible for five hundred thousand deaths every year.[15]

There is also good news. Since peaking in the late 1960s, the death rate from cardiovascular diseases has fallen. In 1999, the mortality rate was less than 40 percent of the rate in 1950.[16] Back then, heart disease was an acute, often fatal condition. After a heart attack, patients were simply sent home to rest and to die. Today doctors are adept at various treatments—clot-busting drugs, tiny balloons to open arteries, bypass surgery—so that heart disease, though still prevalent, is more often chronic than fatal. These advances keep many of the sixty-four million Americans with heart disease alive longer.

In the first stage of heart disease, *angina*, blood flow to the heart is restricted. When blood flow stops, that's a *myocardial infarction*, or *heart attack*. Together, angina and a heart attack are what doctors call *coronary heart disease*. *Arteriosclerosis*, or hardening of the arterial walls, is partly a function of age; with time, the smooth, elastic arterial cells become fibrous and stiff. Arteriosclerosis may be a protective measure to prevent the arteries from expanding under the pressure of blood; veins, which carry blood to the heart at much lower pressure, don't stiffen in this way. When arterial walls become thick and swollen, it's called an *atheroma*; many atheromas are known as *atherosclerosis*. Atheromas, which contain calcium, cholesterol, and fats, may burst, causing blood clots or heart attacks.

The cholesterol hypothesis holds that saturated fats raise cholesterol and cholesterol clogs arteries, but a number of researchers, some of whom belong to a network called the International Committee of Cholesterol Skeptics, are doubtful. "The truth is that the cholesterol theory has never been proven," says Dr. Kilmer McCully, whom I quoted earlier on oxidized cholesterol in powdered eggs. "Elevation of blood cholesterol is a symptom—not a cause—of heart disease." Here is Ravnskov, a leading skeptic and the author of *The Cholesterol Myths*: "When the cholesterol campaign was introduced in Sweden in 1989, I was very surprised. Having followed the scientific literature about cholesterol and cardiovascular disease superficially for years, I could not recall any study showing that high cholesterol was dangerous to the heart, or that any type of dietary fat was more beneficial or harmful than another. I became curious and started to read more systematically. Anyone who reads the literature in this field with an open mind soon discovers that the emperor has no clothes."[17]

At first I thought the skeptics might be few in number, but I found them all over. In 1978, a National Institutes of Health conference held to discuss the drop in death rates from heart attacks since the 1960s was unable to account for the decline by changes in fat and cholesterol consumption or blood cholesterol.[18] Yet this statement got little attention. In 1998, a British National Health Service review found that blood cholesterol alone was a "relatively poor predictor of individual risk."[19] The authors concluded that for the general population, "cholesterol screening is unlikely to reduce mortality and can be misleading or even harmful."

As you might imagine, the cholesterol skeptics have not received a hearty embrace from the medical and pharmaceutical establishment. In Finland, supporters of the anticholesterol campaign belittled Ravnskov's book on television, and then—literally—set the book on fire. When I read *The Cholesterol Myths*, I got excited too, but it didn't put me in the mood to burn books. Quite the opposite: it made me want to buy them. I began to read medical journals and textbooks, and soon I was a skeptic, too.

Does saturated fat raise cholesterol? Not in unhealthy ways. Early studies did show that certain saturated fats, when compared with polyunsaturated oils, raise total cholesterol, but now we know that total cholesterol is a poor predictor of heart disease. In fact, saturated fats raise HDL and polyunsaturated oils lower it. The National Cholesterol Education Program is clear about the virtues of HDL: "the higher, the better." The general effect of saturated fats is to restore a healthy balance of HDL and LDL. Coconut oil, for example, raises HDL if it's low, and lowers LDL if it's high. As we've seen, certain saturated fats (stearic acid in beef and chocolate, and palmitic acid in butter and coconut oil) are good for HDL and LDL ratios.[20] There is abundant evidence from traditional diets to absolve saturated fats. In Nigeria, for example, the Fulani get half their calories from fats, half of which are saturated. Despite what the theory predicts, they have low LDL.[21]

Does high blood cholesterol predict heart disease? In a striking number of cases, the link is weak. Since 1948, researchers have studied the residents of Framingham, Massachusetts, a city near Boston. After a few years, directors of the now famous Framingham Heart Study reported findings that became the bedrock of the cholesterol hypothesis: when they sorted people by low, normal, and high cholesterol, those with high levels had more fatal heart attacks. But almost half the heart attack patients had normal or low cholesterol. In Russia, a twelve-year study of more than sixty-four hundred men found those with low cholesterol had more heart disease.[22] A study in rural China found that neither cholesterol nor LDL was linked to heart disease.[23]

I could cite many other examples—and the cholesterol skeptics do, at length—but the point, I hope, is clear: in Massachusetts, Russia, and China, something other than high cholesterol must be to blame for a large number of heart disease cases.

Cholesterol may be a concern for a relatively small group of people: younger men at high risk of heart disease, such as those who've already had one heart attack. In 1987, the Framingham data showed an association between high cholesterol and mortality for men under forty-seven. But for men older than forty-seven and for all women, there was *no association* between cholesterol and death rates from all causes, including heart disease.[24] According to James Wright of the University of British Columbia, compared with high blood pressure, obesity, diabetes, and smoking, cholesterol is the weakest risk factor for women and heart disease.

The Center for Medical Consumers believes that the heart disease–awareness campaign exaggerates risks for women. One hears that cardiovascular diseases kill almost five hundred thousand women a year in the United States, but nearly 80 percent of heart-related deaths occur in women older than seventy-five. Associate Director Maryann Napoli described what the Framingham researchers found: "Cholesterol was identified as one, but only one, of 240 risk factors that included male baldness, creased ear lobes, and being married to a highly educated woman. Research focused on cholesterol because it is a modifiable risk factor (translation: drug industry opportunity). Though the Framingham Study found a strong association between . . . cholesterol and heart disease only in young and middle-aged men, the entire population was . . . instructed to fear this particular risk factor."

The vast set of data from the prestigious, long-running Framingham study will provide rich research material for years to come. For now, consider this fact. According to Dr. William Castelli, director of the Framingham study, "the more saturated fat one ate, the more cholesterol one ate . . . the lower the person's serum cholesterol."[25] When Castelli made this astonishing admission in 1992, it didn't make news.

Diet First, Then Medication

SUPPOSE YOU WERE A DOCTOR, and the patient sitting before you is a fit woman in her midsixties. According to official guidelines, she has "high" cholesterol of 261 milligrams and "borderline high" LDL of 153 milligrams, but her HDL and triglycerides are great. Current advice from the National Cholesterol Education Program is to lower total cholesterol and LDL aggressively.[26] What should you do?

Some doctors would write a prescription for a statin drug, which blocks the liver from making cholesterol. Statins are the best-selling drug in the United States, worth sixteen billion dollars a year. Pfizer, which makes Lipitor, spends sixty million dollars a year marketing statins to consumers and employs thousands of sales representatives to promote it to doctors.[27] About fifteen million Americans take statins, but under 2004 guidelines, twice that many—thirty-five million people—are candidates. Cardiologists call statins "aspirin for the heart" and joke about putting them in the water supply.

In this not-quite-hypothetical case, the patient happens to be my mother, and I was glad her doctor didn't prescribe a statin. Mom doesn't need to worry about her total cholesterol or her LDL. First, total cholesterol is a poor predictor of heart disease in women and older people. Second, her ratio of total cholesterol to HDL puts her in the "below average" risk category. Third, in women and men over sixty-five, high LDL means longer life.[28]

Statins are highly effective at reducing LDL, and some studies show they can reduce the risk of dying of a heart attack. But some researchers have doubts. Benefits of statins for total mortality—or death from all causes, the gold standard in epidemiology—are small or nonexistent. In 2004, Britain was the first country to approve over-the-counter sales of a statin. The *Lancet* objected, noting that five major trials found that death from all causes was similar with and without statins.[29] "Statins have not been shown to provide an overall mortality benefit," wrote the *Lancet* editors.

Statins may work for a fairly small group. "The people who benefit are middle-aged men who are at high risk or have heart disease," Dr. Beatrice Golomb said. "The benefits do not extend to the elderly or to women." Golomb, who describes herself as "pro-statin," is a medical professor at the University of California and the lead investigator in a large federally financed statin study.

(Diabetics may also benefit from statins, but it seems sensible to treat the most common form, type 2 diabetes, with diet first, because diet causes it.)

As with any treatment, benefits must be weighed against costs. Side effects of statins include muscle weakness, nerve damage, kidney failure, liver damage, and memory loss. A rare but serious side effect is the potentially fatal muscle-wasting disorder rhabdomyolysis. In 2001 a statin linked to thirty-one rhabdomyolysis deaths was withdrawn. Statins deplete coenzyme Q_{10} an antioxidant found in fish, pork, heart, and liver. Used to prevent and treat heart disease in the United States and Japan, CoQ_{10} prevents LDL from being oxidized.[30] "The first thing I do with new heart patients," says cardiologist Dr. Peter Langsjoen, who has reviewed many studies on CoQ_{10}, "is take them off statins."[31]

What constitutes healthy cholesterol levels is also a matter of debate. The National Cholesterol Education Program says total cholesterol under 200 milligrams is "desirable." But this target is not particularly useful. First, "total cholesterol" is not really cholesterol at all, but a composite number equal to HDL, LDL, and 20 percent of triglycerides. We now know that total cholesterol does not predict heart disease. Despite the bad press, "high LDL" is a poor predictor, too. Other readings such as triglycerides, blood sugar, and C-Reactive Protein (CRP) are more useful.

Some doctors think it's unwise to reduce cholesterol at all costs. Attention has focused on "the supposed danger" of high blood cholesterol for fifty years, says Barry Groves, a British researcher on obesity, diabetes, and heart disease, while "the dangers of low blood cholesterol levels have largely been ignored."[32] Older people, for example, benefit from high cholesterol. Death rates in the elderly from all causes, including heart disease, are greater with low cholesterol.[33] Thus the *Lancet* advises doctors to be "cautious" about reducing cholesterol in people over sixty-five.[34]

Low cholesterol is linked to respiratory disease, HIV, depression, and death by violence or suicide. Low cholesterol is also associated with another serious cardiovascular disease: stroke.[35]

Cholesterol protects against infection, a well-known risk factor for heart disease. Infection leads to inflammation, which appears in the arterial walls of heart disease patients with normal cholesterol. A good measure of inflammation is CRP, a risk factor for heart disease.[36] Women with high CRP and healthy cholesterol have twice as many heart attacks.[37] Inflammation is caused by excess omega-6 fats, smoking, and gum disease, another risk factor for heart disease. Exercise reduces both inflammation and CRP, which is produced in fat cells.

Clearly, there is much more to learn from the lab than just our LDL and HDL levels. Heart disease has many causes. That means there are no simple answers in diagnosis, prevention, and treatment. On the positive side, there are potentially many cures. For example, if my mother wanted to lower her LDL without taking drugs, she could eat more fish. Omega-3 fats reduce LDL, raise HDL, lower triglycerides, prevent clots, reduce blood pressure, and fight inflammation. Fish is powerful stuff—and it has no side effects.

Another nutritional approach to reducing LDL (if it worries you) is eating soy, almonds, oats, barley, okra, and eggplant. Dubbed the *portfolio diet*, this regimen compares favorably with statins in lowering LDL.[38] University of Toronto researchers gave people with high cholesterol three treatments: one group ate a diet "very low" in saturated fat, the second ate the portfolio diet, and the third took statins. The statin treatment and the portfolio diet were equally good, each reducing LDL by about 30 percent. The diet low in saturated fat was the least effective, reducing LDL by only 8 percent. (The low-saturated fat diet, I noted, was also heavy on industrial foods: sunflower oil, fat-free cheese, egg substitutes, liquid egg whites, and "light" margarine.)

How does the portfolio diet work? Almonds are rich in monounsaturated fat, which lowers LDL. Soy isoflavones lower LDL. The viscous fiber in whole grains, okra, and eggplant also lowers LDL, perhaps by mopping up bile acid, which forces the liver to use up cholesterol to make more bile acid. The title of the editorial to accompany this small but promising study in the *Journal of the American Medical Association* was clear enough: "Diet First, Then Medication."

A Disease of Deficiency

> Kilmer McCully has indeed led a revolution because his work . . . has provided powerful evidence that nutritional deficiencies are an important cause of heart disease. Not surprisingly, this notion encountered great resistance . . . This is also the story of a personal struggle by a brilliant physician against a powerful and rigid scientific establishment.
>
> —Dr. Walter Willett, Harvard School of Public Health

IN 1968, KILMER MCCULLY was a young pathologist studying inherited diseases at Massachusetts General Hospital in Boston. One day, pediatricians told McCully about an eight-year-old boy who had died of a stroke at the same hospital in 1933. The case was unusual enough to be written up in the *New England Journal of Medicine*, and it made McCully curious. When he tracked down the original autopsy slides, he saw the severe arteriosclerosis diagnosed by the pathologist on the boy's death thirty-five years before.

The boy had a rare genetic disease called homocystinuria, which is caused by faulty B vitamin metabolism and named for homocysteine, an amino acid that appears in the urine. Other symptoms include long limbs, mild mental retardation, and severe arteriosclerosis. Children with homocystinuria die of conditions one associates with old age: blood clots, heart attack, stroke. There is no cure, but high doses of vitamin B_6 help relieve symptoms in about half of patients.

McCully happened to be familiar with homocysteine and cholesterol metabolism.[39] In 1968, the leading theory of arteriosclerosis was that cholesterol attacked the arteries. But McCully didn't believe cholesterol caused the damage he saw in this case. If cholesterol caused arteriosclerosis, why was there no cholesterol in this boy's arteries? Mulling it over, McCully recalled animal studies linking deficiency of B vitamins and folic acid to arteriosclerosis, and he reflected on the cause of homocystinuria: faulty B vitamin metabolism. After many sleepless nights, his eureka moment came: McCully realized that excess homocysteine due to lack of B vitamins and folic acid caused arteriosclerosis. Cholesterol did not.

In 1969, McCully described his hypothesis about arteriosclerosis in the *American Journal of Pathology* and proposed a simple treatment: folic acid and B vitamins to keep homocysteine down. At first, this alternative theory of arteriosclerosis was big news, and scientists all over the world asked for copies of the article. In 1970, the hospital praised his work as an example of "the unpredictable, important contributions which can come when an imaginative, skilled worker is given free reign to follow his findings."

But the warm reception was brief. The cholesterol hypothesis was still the establishment view; in 1968, experts had decreed that 300 milligrams of dietary cholesterol daily was the "safe" upper limit. As news spread of this apparent threat to the cholesterol theory, the medical world shunned McCully. He lost his research funding and his posts at Harvard and Massachusetts General Hospital. He went jobless for two years.

Now, more than thirty-five years later, McCully is the chief of pathology at the Veterans Affairs Medical Center in Boston, and he treats the affair as a backhanded compliment. "If what I had discovered was unimportant, no one would have cared," McCully told me brightly.[40] He can afford to be magnanimous, because today the role of homocysteine is widely accepted. The landmark Physicians' Health Study on diet and heart disease found that male doctors with high homocysteine were three times more likely to have a heart attack than those with normal levels. In the large and prestigious Nurses' Health Study, women who ate the least folic acid and vitamin B_6 had the highest heart-related death rates. The famous Framingham Heart Study also linked homocysteine to heart disease. McCully's rehabilitation is complete. He is known as the "father of homocysteine."

About twenty human trials examining homocysteine are under way all over the world. McCully is supervising the Homocysteine Study, a national clinical trial of two thousand veterans sponsored by the U.S. Department of Veterans Affairs, in which people with kidney failure—a risk factor for heart disease—are taking a placebo or large doses of folic acid and vitamins B_6 and B_{12}.

B VITAMINS AND FOLIC ACID IN THE HOMOCYSTEINE STUDY

Note the large vitamin doses in the Homocysteine Study (HOST). Folic acid and B vitamins are perfectly safe.

	*RDA**	*Ideal RDA†*	*Daily dose in HOST*
Vitamin B_6	2 mg	3–3.5 mg	100 mg
Vitamin B_{12}	6 mcg	5–15 mcg	2,000 mcg
Folic acid	400 mcg	400 mcg	40,000 mcg

* Recommended Daily Allowance (RDA)

† According to Kilmer McCully, *The Heart Revolution*

The normal role of homocysteine is to control growth and support tissue formation, but in excess, it damages the cells of arterial walls, destroys the elasticity of the artery, and contributes to calcification of plaques. Vitamins help by reducing homocysteine. Folic acid and vitamin B_{12} convert it to harmless methionine, and vitamin B_6 converts it to cysteine, which is excreted. Less well known nutrients betaine and choline also reduce homocysteine.

The actions of homocysteine fit with what we know about heart disease. It raises triglycerides and forms oxidized LDL, which causes arteriosclerosis.[41] Homocysteine travels on LDL, which explains the high LDL seen in some people with heart disease. In addition to diet, many other factors—old age, menopause, smoking, diabetes, lack of exercise, being male, high blood pressure—raise homocysteine, and every one is linked to heart disease. "All along, it was homocysteine causing the damage," writes McCully, "while cholesterol was getting the blame."

A popular parlor game in cholesterol circles is solving the mystery known as the French Paradox. Why do the French have low rates of heart disease despite relatively high blood cholesterol and a diet rich in saturated fats? The French Paradox is only paradoxical if you believe that natural saturated fats cause heart disease, of course. But let's pretend they do for the moment. Perhaps red wine is the answer, or smaller portions.

McCully believes the key to the mystery is the pâté, sautéed calves' liver, and sweetbreads the French are so fond of. Liver and organ meats are superlative sources of folic acid and B vitamins, which keep homocysteine levels low. Homocysteine also explains why people from Papua New Guinea to Nigeria can eat liberal amounts of saturated fat and yet escape heart disease—another paradox for the conventional wisdom. Traditional diets are low in white flour and sugar (which deplete B vitamins) and rich in meat, liver, fish, whole grains, and green vegetables, all of which are good sources of folic acid and B vitamins.

WHAT TO EAT TO KEEP HOMOCYSTEINE LOW

Folic acid, vitamins B_6 and B_{12}, betaine, and choline reduce homocysteine. Note that B_{12} is found only in animal foods.

B_{12}	*B_6*	*Folic acid*	*Betaine*	*Choline*
Fish	Fish	Liver	Eggs	Eggs
Meat	Meat	Leafy greens	Liver	Meat
Liver	Poultry	Citrus	Beets	Wheat germ
Dairy	Liver	Whole grains		
Clams	Whole grains	Peas		
Oysters	Peas	Beans		
	Nuts	Nuts		
	Broccoli			
	Lentils			
	Leafy greens			
	Sweet potatoes			
	Winter squash			
	Bananas			

To keep homocysteine levels healthy, eat beef, liver, oysters, eggs, whole grains, and green vegetables. Remember that vitamin B_{12} is found only in animal foods, especially salmon, tuna, cheese, eggs, liver, beef, and lamb. Also, nutrients are lost when food is processed. About 80 percent of folic acid disappears when whole wheat flour is milled into white flour, and vitamin B_6 is easily damaged by heat. Thus canned tuna contains half as much B_6 as fresh tuna. Vitamin B_{12} is more robust to heat, but microwaves damage nutrients much more than conventional heat.

McCully was not the first to blame industrial foods for heart disease, but his discovery about homocysteine was a giant leap forward in our understanding of how, exactly, refined foods damage the arteries. "The first case of heart disease as it is known today was reported in 1912, the second in 1919, and since then it has developed into a major killer," wrote Adelle Davis in *Let's Get Well*. "The obvious change has been the ever-increasing consumption of refined foods and hydrogenated fats. The populations of the world living today on unrefined foods, in which nature packages with her fats all the nutrients needed to utilize them, do not develop heart disease." She was writing in 1965. More than forty years later, Adelle Davis's books are still worth reading. Even more remarkable, her work is cutting edge.

BEYOND CHOLESTEROL

What Causes Heart Disease

- Deficiency of any of the following: omega-3 fats; folic acid, vitamins B_6 and B_{12}; antioxidants, including CoQ_{10} and vitamins C and E
- Excess omega-6 fats (polyunsaturated vegetable oils)
- Inflammation (from infection and excess corn oil)
- Oxidized cholesterol (from free radicals in the body and powdered eggs and milk)
- Sugar
- Trans fats (hydrogenated oils)

A Few Risk Factors

- Age (84 percent of people who die of heart disease are sixty-five or older)
- Excess weight, particularly belly fat
- Sedentary lifestyle
- Diabetes (also metabolic syndrome, or prediabetes)
- Family history of heart disease

10

The Omnivore's Dilemma

IN THE EARLY 1970S, my father's parents came to visit us in Buffalo, New York, en route to Yugoslavia. Then, as now, we ate simple food, always made from scratch: some protein, whole grains, vegetables, a green salad. Sugar was a treat. As they left, my grandfather said cheerfully, "Let's hope there's dessert in Yugoslavia!"

It is said that every household resembles a small nation-state. If so, each family has its Department of Health and its food and cooking policies. In our house, my mother (like most mothers) wrote the law. Like most daughters, I left home, founded a new colony of sorts, and wrote my own (vegan and vegetarian) laws. When that turned out badly, I was happy to come home to the foods I'd grown up eating, but I also wanted to know what science had to say about them. Now I am satisfied that butter and eggs are good for you.

It is not easy to decide what to eat. There are virtually no limits today. We are not like foragers, who found a beehive dripping with honey only now and then; we are not like the babies in the Clara Davis experiments, who could choose only from nutritious foods. And things move fast. In the modern food industry, novelty and technical wizardry are the rule. In the United States, ten thousand new processed foods come on the market each year, and it seems a new diet is always climbing the best-seller list. Unlike industrial food, real food is fundamentally conservative. It is the food you already know: roast chicken, tomato salad with olive oil, creamed spinach, sourdough bread, peach ice cream. To me, that's a relief. When you rule out industrial foods altogether, it does simplify things a bit.

The quest for the right diet is not a modern conundrum. It is not merely the result of unprecedented variety and abundance or even of the profusion of contradictory nutritional advice. On the contrary, our search for the right food is as old as eating itself. Since prehistoric times, every human has asked: *what's for dinner?*

Culture undoubtedly plays a role in how we decide what to eat. Hindus don't eat cows, for example. But culture is a minor determinant compared with nutritional needs, which traditionally trump all other factors. What will nourish the body for a day's labor, through a long winter, or to recover from an infection? Survival alone is not enough. For men as well as women, food must also be adequate to ensure fertility. For most creatures, nutrition is simple: instinct rules. Insect or mammal, herbivore or carnivore, the menu is typically short. Parsnip worms eat parsnip seeds, ladybugs eat aphids, koala bears eat eucalyptus leaves, zebras eat grass, and lions eat zebras. But we are omnivores. We can and will eat anything.

Omnivores are highly adaptable and humans especially so. That's why we occupy not one ecological niche but many, from frozen tundra to moist forest to scorched desert. This is a singular achievement; no other species lives in all the major habitats. A penchant for trying new foods in new situations was key to the success of all the *Homo* tribes, including ours. "When the eucalyptus trees all die in a given place, so do all the koalas," writes Richard Manning, "but omnivores have options."

Along with these options comes a unique problem, namely, that not everything that looks like food is edible and some things might be poisonous. In 1976, the psychologist Paul Rozin called this the *omnivore's dilemma.* One eucalyptus tree meets all the nutritional needs of a hungry koala, but an omnivore must successfully balance curiosity and caution to survive. Various tactics come in handy. As social animals, we pass the word along that this berry or that insect is to be eaten or avoided. Contemporary hunter-gatherers without formal education in botany or zoology can identify hundreds of plant and animal species and many details about their medicinal or toxic properties, life cycles, habitat, and habits. The Harvard psychologist Steven Pinker calls this *intuitive biology,* and it is surely the product of the omnivore's quandary. Omnivores also avoid things that smell rotten, and only nibble at unfamiliar foods. Researchers describe another tactic as the "poisoned partner effect." If a rat smelling of a particular food is looking poorly, other rats will avoid that food.

Even so, omnivores do get things wrong, especially in new situations, and suffer for it. When Americans settled west of the Appalachians in the 1800s, people began to get "milk sickness," which caused weakness, nausea, thirst, foul breath, and finally, death. In certain Indiana and Ohio counties, the illness was rampant. It was noticeable that where people were dying, cattle with similar symptoms got the "trembles." The twin epidemics aroused the curiosity of an Illinois midwife, Anna Pierce, who asked a local Shawnee woman for advice. The woman led her directly to white snakeroot, a plant that caused the trembles in cows and poisoned the milk. The active compound of snakeroot—tremetol—was not identified until 1928. One doctor who doubted that Pierce had found the cause of milk sickness ate snakeroot to prove her wrong; he promptly died.

In modern life, the risk of unintentional poisoning is greatly reduced. We don't have to guess which foods might make us sick because the food supply is no longer wild. Botany is now a formal body of knowledge, scientifically tested. My parents taught me that rhubarb leaves contain toxic oxalic acid, while the stems make great pie; they learned that from books, not at the knee of the local wise woman. But the modern omnivore is not out of the woods yet. The risk of nutritional imbalance is great. Rozin writes: "A koala that eats only eucalyptus leaves has no such risk; it is adapted to survive on the nutrients eucalyptus has to offer. Similarly, a lion rarely risks imbalance, because the zebras it eats already contain the range of nutrients it needs. But the generalist happens upon many potential foods that have nutritive value, but are not complete nutrients. Appropriate combinations of foods must be selected."

There's the rub. Unlike lions and other specialists, we have to think about which foods are nourishing, and in this respect, life is more confusing than ever. Modern humans face a vast choice of food, far beyond what was ever available before in both variety and quantity. Although traditional diets vary widely, in any given place, humans always ate a limited menu of local, seasonal foods.

Together, technology and migration have produced an unprecedented profusion of food. Freezing, canning, pasteurization, and other technologies extend the shelf life of perishable foods. Global trade has expanded variety beyond the imagination of any hunter-gatherer. The coffee, tea, spice, and olive oil trades are thousands of years old, but even this ancient commerce is recent in evolutionary time. The scale of modern trade is astounding. When there is snow on the ground, we can eat sweet corn and tomatoes; in cold climates, mangos and pineapples are easy to come by; in most American towns, Italian olive oil, Chilean grapes, and Thai shrimp are not luxuries but staples. Perhaps the most profound contribution of technology is the creation of truly new foods such as canola oil and margarine.

As exotic foods have circled the globe, so have people. Migration has loosened, if not severed, the bonds between people and their traditional foods. For most of human history, a child ate what her parents ate: yogurt in Turkey, miso soup in Japan, cheese in the Swiss Alps. Today, the foods of every culture, from hummus to tortillas, mingle in restaurants, shops, and markets. The United States, a land of immigrants, is particularly diverse—and apt to slough off tradition—but something similar occurs in most wealthy nations: the typical diet is not the traditional one. The modern omnivore's dilemma is acute.

THE OMNIVORE'S FEAST—WHAT'S FOR DINNER?

- Eat generous amounts of fresh fruits and vegetables daily
- Eat wild fish and seafood often
- Eat meat, game, poultry, and eggs from wild, pastured, and grass-fed animals often
- Eat full-fat dairy foods, ideally raw and unhomogenized from grass-fed cows, often
- Eat only traditional fats, including butter, lard, poultry fat, coconut oil, and olive oil
- Eat whole grains and legumes
- Eat cultured and fermented foods such as yogurt, sauerkraut, miso, and sourdough bread
- Eat unrefined sweeteners such as raw honey, evaporated cane juice, and pure maple syrup in moderation

For three million years, we were skilled fishermen and hunters, able to kill giant animals such as wooly mammoths and fast ones such as wild horses, not to mention lions, sloths, bears, moose, giant lemurs, and camels. We hunted with a powerful combination of tools unique in the animal world: sharp spears, binocular vision, hand-eye coordination, and teamwork. We filled up on fish and game when we could, and in between we made do with every berry, tuber, and insect we could find. This dietary strategy—mostly predator, part forager—was simple and effective.

Then, in the blink of an evolutionary eye, something catastrophic happened. About thirty-five thousand years ago, the megafauna (big game) dwindled and then disappeared. "They became extinct in every habitat without exception," writes the historian Jared Diamond, "from deserts to cold rain forest and tropical rain forest." We humans were the main predator of these wild animals, which had thrived for tens of millions of years before we arrived. Until recently the suggestion that we killed them off—the "overkill hypothesis"—was ridiculed. Now most scientists agree that the big game were not doomed by an ice age or drought, but by spears and clubs.

Having depleted our chief source of nutrition, we did what only omnivores can do. We went looking for other foods to eat. We hunted less big game and began, gradually, to domesticate smaller wild animals for meat and milk. We foraged more and began to nurture wild crops like yams. The result was amazing variety in our diet. When an Iron Age man slipped into a peat bog in Denmark twenty-two hundred years ago, his stomach held the remains of sixty species of plants. Our brains are wired and our bodies are built to hunt and gather. Hunger is our motivation, variety is the result, and health is our reward.

Perhaps this explains my urge to forage. At the farm, I enjoy nothing more than picking vegetables for dinner, finding nettles behind the barn, or cutting watercress from the footbridge over the creek. Browsing the farmers' market always makes me happy. Even rummaging in the fridge in search of inspiration for dinner is a little adventure.

Variety is the hallmark of the human diet and its greatest pleasure. At my house, there may be a dozen different foods—from beef to bacon, olive oil to butter, kohlrabi to zucchini—at just one meal. I am not ambitious enough to put sixty vegetables, much less sixty species, on the dinner table, but when I am shopping for food or cooking dinner, I try to remember the rich array of life in the last supper of the Iron Age man, and I feel lucky to be an omnivore, blessed with a thousand ways to eat well and be well.

Where to Find Real Food

Local Foods

Local food is sold in all kinds of venues. These two national sites cover all the options, from farmers' markets to farm stands and farm shares.
www.foodroutes.org
www.localharvest.org

American Farmers' Markets
Find your local farmers' market. The USDA keeps a reasonably comprehensive list of farmers' markets in the United States.
www.ams.usda.gov/farmersmarkets

British Farmers' Markets
In London: www.lfm.org.uk
FARMA lists farmers' markets in the United Kingdom.
www.farma.org.uk

American Farm Shares or Community-Supported Agriculture
Buy a farm share and get a weekly delivery of local foods all season. Most farm shares include produce and flowers; some add meat, dairy, poultry, and eggs.
www.nal.usda.gov/afsic/csa

Grass-Fed and Pastured Meat, Dairy, Poultry, Eggs, and Game

Jo Robinson, author of *Pasture Perfect*, provides excellent information on the benefits of grass-fed meat, dairy, eggs, poultry, and game, and posts an extensive directory of foods.
www.eatwild.com

Niman Ranch is a network of several hundred independent farmers and ranchers who raise traditional beef, lamb, and pork. Look for *lardo*, ham, bacon, and other cured meats without nitrites.
www.nimanranch.com or 510-808-0340

In Virginia, Buffalo Hunter Meats sells American bison, grass-fed beef, pastured pork and poultry, and rabbit. Try the jerky and bacon.
www.buffalohuntermeats.com or 540-727-8590

Mercola, a natural foods and nutrition Web site, sells grass-fed, hormone- and antibiotic-free bison; wild Alaskan salmon; grass-fed, organic, and raw milk cheese.
www.mercola.com

The Campaign for Real Milk describes raw milk laws in each state and will lead you to buying clubs and cow shares for raw milk, butter, cream, yogurt, and cheese.
www.realmilk.com

Organic Pastures Dairy sells organic, grass-fed raw milk, cheese, and butter in California. It ships raw dairy foods frozen, exclusively for feeding pets (nod, wink).
www.organicpastures.com or 877-729-6455

Wild and Farmed Fish and Seafood

All Alaskan salmon is wild. Because the state banned fish farming, wild salmon and other fish are abundant in Alaska's clean, icy waters. The best fish is "frozen at sea" and vacuum packed. The following fishing boats, fishing co-ops, and purveyors sell wild salmon, halibut, sablefish, tuna, and other seafood from the Pacific Northwest.

Cape Cleare Fishery, www.capecleare.com or 360-385-7486
Dungeness Seaworks, www.freshfrozenfish.com
Marbled Chinook Salmon, www.marbledsalmon.com
Prime Select Seafood, www.pssifish.com or 888-870-7292
Vital Choice, www.vitalchoice.com or 800-608-4825
Troll-caught Albacore Tuna, www.albatuna.com

Fish Oil

The nanny was right. Cod liver oil is the most valuable fish oil supplement because it contains vitamins A and D along with omega-3 fats. All cod liver oil is refined to some degree, which reduces vitamins. Most manufacturers add synthetic vitamins back. According to an article by David Wetzel in the Fall 2005 issue of *Wise Traditions*, the brands listed below use only natural vitamin A and D. Some are flavored with mint, cinnamon, or citrus. (Nannies served cod liver oil in orange juice, another good method.) If you don't care for cod liver oil, try wild salmon oil capsules from Vital Choice.

Dr. Ron's Ultra-Pure, www.drrons.com or 877-472-8701
Green Pastures, www.greenpasture.org or 402-338-5551
Radiant Life, www.radiantlifecatalog.com or 888-593-8333
Vital Choice, www.vitalchoice.com or 800-608-4825

Traditional American Corn, Wheat, and Rice

Anson Mills sells organic whole heirloom seed corn, wheat, and Carolina gold rice grown on farms in Georgia, Virginia, and the Carolinas. Grits and biscuit flour are cold-milled to preserve flavor and nutrients. Carolina gold and white rice are buffered and milled with colonial methods.
www.ansonmills.com or 803-467-4122

Hoppin' John Taylor sells whole-grain grits, cornmeal, and corn flour ground from heirloom Appalachian dent corn grown with ecological methods in Georgia. A high-fat variety, the corn is grown above twenty-five hundred feet (to reduce pest, mold, and mildew damage), left to dry fully in the field, and then ground between blue granite stones. The ground corn is never sifted, which leaves the bran, fat, and flavor intact. An expert on southern foods, Taylor is the author of several cookbooks, including *Hoppin' John's Lowcountry Cooking*.
www.hoppinjohns.com or 800-828-4412

Chocolate

Scharffen Berger makes chocolate in small batches with vintage European equipment and traditional methods. The unsweetened chocolate and cacao nibs are superb.
www.scharffenberger.com or 800-930-4528

Chocosphere sells many international chocolates. I like the French Pralus, British Green & Black's, and Grenada.
www.chocosphere.com or 877-992-4626

Sweeteners

Find local raw honey and pure maple syrup at farmers' markets, farm stands, and health food stores. For mail order, try these:

Deep Mountain Maple Syrup sells pure maple syrup and pure maple sugar made with traditional methods in West Glover, Vermont.
www.deepmountainmaple.com or 802-525-4162

Tropical Traditions and the Grain and Salt Society sell organic whole sugar.
www.tropicaltraditions.com or 866-311-2626
www.celticseasalt.com or 800-867-7528

Various Traditional Foods

Radiant Life sells traditional foods based on the research of Weston Price, including grass-fed, raw butter, unrefined sea salt, unfiltered olive oil, and cod-liver oil.
www.radiantlifecatalog.com or 888-593-8333

Members of the Weston A. Price Foundation receive a newsletter, *Wise Traditions*. The classified section features local grass-fed and pastured meat, poultry, eggs, and dairy, and other traditional foods such as coconut oil and salmon roe.
www.westonaprice.org or 202-363-4394

The Grain and Salt Society sells traditional foods, including unrefined sea salt, wild salmon, and fermented foods.
www.celticseasalt.com or 800-867-7528

Traditional Soy Foods

You will find miso, natto, and tempeh in health food stores, good grocery stores, and Asian markets. Clearspring is a good brand of organic and fermented Asian foods.

Coconut Oil

Tropical Traditions sells wet-milled, virgin coconut oil and a rich coconut cream from small organic farms in the Philippines. It also sells coconut soap and skin cream.
www.tropicaltraditions.com or 866-311-2626

Unrefined Salt

Only unrefined sea salt contains the essential trace elements. Saltworks offers unrefined salts from all over the world. Real Salt sells unrefined salt from ancient Utah salt mines. (Originally—in the Jurassic era—it *was* sea salt.) Celtic is another good brand.
www.saltworks.us or 800-353-7258
www.realsalt.com or 800-367-7258
www.celticseasalt.com or 800-867-7258

Breast-Feeding and Infant Formula

For information and encouragement about breast-feeding, contact La Leche League.
www.lalecheleague.org or 847-519-7730

If you cannot feed your baby with breast milk, find a recipe for the next best thing at www.westonaprice.org. Many of the ingredients can be found at www.radiantlife.com.

Further Reading and Resources

Further Reading

All these books are for the general reader. Most are less famous than they should be. Together, they represent a mountain of good sense on food, cooking, diet, health, and agriculture. Every one ought to be a best seller.

Food and Cooking

Appetite, Nigel Slater
An English home cook with a taste for simple things, Slater is my favorite food writer. *Appetite* is a bible for daily home cooking, teaching you how to cook by loose recipes and general principles.

The Complete Dairy Foods Cookbook, Annie Proulx and Lew Nichols
This wonderful book on homemade dairy is sadly out of print and worth buying used.

Good Fat, Fran McCullough
A cookbook that makes sense of real and industrial fats.

The Grassfed Gourmet Cookbook, Shannon Hayes
Cooking grass-fed beef properly takes some practice. Get it here.

Last Chance to Eat: The Fate of Taste in a Fast Food World, Gina Mallet

A lyrical memoir told via the fate of four foods—eggs, fish, beef, raw milk cheese—with lots of facts for the serious and curious.

Nourishing Traditions, Sally Fallon and Mary Enig
A kitchen bible, with all the recipes you need, plus tons of useful information on traditional food.

On Food and Cooking: The Science and Lore of the Kitchen, Harold McGee
McGee is indispensable on the science of the kitchen. You will refer to him often.

The Primal Feast: Food, Sex, Foraging, and Love, Susan Allport
Allport writes with the naturalist's eye on the human omnivore, why women hoard and share food, how farming caused our health to decline, food cravings, and more.

The Whole Beast, Fergus Henderson
Henderson is the chef at St. John, a superb London restaurant dedicated to the whole beast, from meat to feet, cheek to marrow.

Health and Diet

The Cholesterol Myths: Exposing the Fallacy That Cholesteral and Saturated Fat Cause Heart Disease, Uffe Ravnskov
If you know someone who's afraid to eat butter and eggs, this book will do the trick. See www.thincs.org.

The Healing Miracles of Coconut Oil, Bruce Fife
If you read this slim book and are still unsure about *eating* coconut oil, it will, I hope, at least persuade you to use it on your skin. I swear by pure coconut oil soap and lotion from Tropical Traditions. (See "Where to Find Real Food," page 281.)

The Heart Revolution: The Extraordinary Discovery That Finally Laid the Cholesterol Myth to Rest and Put Good Food Back on the Table, Kilmer McCully and Martha McCully
This readable paperback explains why cholesterol is not the enemy and how real food rich in B vitamins prevents heart disease.

The Omega-3 Connection: The Ground-Breaking Anti-Depression and Diet Program, Andrew Stoll
Fish prevents obesity, diabetes, heart disease, and depression.

The Paleo Diet: Lose Weight and Get Healthy Eating the Food You Were Designed to Eat, Loren Cordain
Cordain recommends we eat like hunter-gatherers. His research on obesity, diabetes, and heart disease is very useful.
See www.thepaleodiet.com.

Farming

Against the Grain: How Agriculture Has Hijacked Civilization, Richard Manning
An unforgettable account of the triumph of cereal crops in agriculture.

Keeping a Family Cow, Joann S. Grohman
An expert in cow and human nutrition, Grohman writes for (very) small dairy farmers, but anyone who cares about milk will be fascinated. Buy her book at www.real-food.com.

The Omnivore's Dilemma: A Natural History of Four Meals, Michael Pollan
Pollan is America's most talented writer on food and agriculture. For recent writings, try www.michaelpollan.com.

Pasture Perfect: The Far-Reaching Benefits of Choosing Meat, Eggs, and Dairy Products from Grass-Fed Animals, Jo Robinson
Robinson is the best exponent of the benefits of grass-fed and pastured foods. See www.eatwild.com.

Salad Bar Beef, Joel Salatin
Salatin is America's most famous grass farmer. This compelling primer on grass-fed beef is for farmers, but anyone will appreciate it.

Organizations

Traditional Foods

The International Network of Cholesterol Skeptics (THINCS)
A loose affiliation of scientists, doctors, and other researchers who

doubt the cholesterol hypothesis of heart disease. Says the founder, Uffe Ravnskov: "Members represent different views about the causation of atherosclerosis and cardiovascular disease. Some conflict with others, but this is a normal part of science. What we all oppose is that animal fat and high cholesterol play a role. The aim is to inform our colleagues and the public that this idea is not supported by scientific evidence; in fact, for many years a huge number of scientific studies have directly contradicted it."
www.thincs.org

Price-Pottenger Nutrition Foundation
Dedicated to the work of Dr. Francis Pottenger, famous for his experiments with raw milk and cats, and to Weston Price, the PPNF offers a newsletter and a library of research about health and nutrition.
www.price-pottenger.org

Slow Food
An international organization founded in Italy with members all over the world, Slow Food protects "the pleasures of the table from the homogenization of modern fast food." Join your local chapter to meet like-minded people and to find local, traditional, and artisanal foods.
www.slowfood.com or www.slowfoodusa.org

Weston A. Price Foundation
Dedicated to the work of Weston Price, this membership organization campaigns for traditional foods, publishes a newsletter on nutrition and disease, and encourages people to buy real food in season from independent, local farmers.
www.westonaprice.org

Sustainable Agriculture

Glynwood Center
Glynwood's Agricultural Initiative promotes local and traditional foods, with an emphasis on small farmers, financially viable farms, scenic habitats, and diverse wildlife.
www.glynwood.org

Institute for Agriculture and Trade Policy
IATP works for environmentally sound and financially viable rural and trade policies.
www.iatp.org

National Campaign for Sustainable Agriculture
An alliance of groups promoting ecological farm policies.
www.sustainableagriculture.net

Movies

The Future of Food
A smart, thorough, and moving documentary on the threat of genetic engineering to small farmers, biodiversity, ecology, and food security for entire nations. Buy the DVD.
www.thefutureoffood.com

The Meatrix
A spoof on the hit film *The Matrix, The Meatrix* is a four-minute flash animation skewering factory farming. Ten million people have seen it. You're next.
www.themeatrix.com

The Real Dirt on Farmer John
A third-generation Illinois farmer turns combines into farm shares.
www.therealdirt.net

Super Size Me
Morgan Spurlock ate industrial foods for thirty days and wrecked his health. Rent the PG version for any kid you love.
www.supersizeme.com

Clothing and Accessories

FoodGoods designs beautiful T-shirts, tote bags, and aprons with amusing slogans about traditional and local foods.
www.foodgoods.com

Notes

1. I Grow Up on Real Food, Lose My Way, and Come Home Again

1. To calculate your BMI, see www.nhlbisupport.com/bmi.
2. William R. Leonard, "Food for Thought," *Scientific American* 13, no. 2 (2003; updated from December 2002 issue).
3. Talk by Michel Odent attended by the author. *Midwifery Today* conference, Philadelphia, March 18, 2004.
4. Lindsay Allen spoke at the 2005 meeting of the American Association for the Advancement of Science.
5. Some vitamin B_{12} is produced by microorganisms in fermentation. Yeast and beer, for example, contain vitamin B_{12} made by these tiny animals. A small quantity of B_{12} prevents deficiency.
6. A. P. Simopoulos, "The Importance of the Ratio of Omega-6/Omega-3 Essential Fatty Acids," *Biomedicine and Pharmacotherapy* 56, no. 8 (2002): 453.
7. Andrew L. Stoll, *The Omega-3 Connection: The Ground-Breaking Anti-Depression and Diet Program* (New York: Fireside, 2001), 92.
8. Anthony Colpo, "LDL Cholesterol: 'Bad' Cholesterol, or Bad Science?" *Journal of American Physicians and Surgeons* 10, no. 3 (2005).
9. N. Schupf et al., "Relationship Between Plasma Lipids and All-Cause Mortality in Non-Demented Elderly," *Journal of the American Geriatrics Society 53* (2005) 219–229.
10. "Malignant Medical Myths About Heart Disease," a talk given on November 13, 2005, by Joel Kauffman attended by the author at the Weston A. Price Foundation Conference in Chantilly, Virginia. See also the chapter on cholesterol from Kauffman's book *Malignant Medical Myths*.
11. Leonard, "Food for Thought."

2. *Real Milk, Butter, and Cheese*

1. A. P. Simopoulos, "The Importance of the Ratio of Omega-6/Omega-3 Essential Fatty Acids," *Biomedicine and Pharmacotherapy* 56, no. 8 (2002): 453.
2. Mary Enig, *Know Your Fats: The Complete Primer for Understanding the Nutrition of Fats, Oils, and Cholesterol* (Silver Spring, MD: Bethesda Press, 2000), 57.
3. R. L. Duyff and the American Dietetic Association, *American Dietetic Association Complete Food and Nutrition Guide*, 2nd ed. (Hoboken, NJ: John Wiley, 2002), 65.
4. The antibodies are known as immunoglobulins. The other four are IgG, IgM, IgD, and IgE.
5. Enig, *Know Your Fats*, 189; and R. Uauy, C. E. Mize, and C. Castillo-Duran, "Fat Intake During Childhood: Metabolic Responses and Effects on Growth," *American Journal of Clinical Nutrition* 72 (2000): S1354–60.
6. For a recipe, see Sally Fallon and Mary Enig, *Nourishing Traditions*, revised 2nd ed. (Washington, DC: NewTrends, 2001) or www.westonaprice.org.
7. J. M. Neeson, *Commoners: Common Rights, Enclosure and Social Change in England, 1700 to 1820* (Cambridge: Cambridge University Press, 1993), 11.
8. Thokild Kjaergaard, *The Danish Revolution, 1500–1800: An Ecohistorical Interpretation*, trans. David Hohnen (Cambridge: Cambridge University Press, 1994), 162–63.
9. Interview with the author on May 6, 2004, prompted by Grout's review of Grohman's book, posted on www.amazon.com on March 23, 2004.
10. Robert Cohen, *Milk: The Deadly Poison* (Englewood Cliffs, NJ: Argus, 1997), 100–101.
11. Albano Beja-Pereira et al., "Gene-Culture Coevolution Between Cattle Milk Protein Genes and Human Lactase Genes," *Nature Genetics*, published online November 23, 2003.
12. Uffe Ravnskov, *The Cholesterol Myths: Exposing the Fallacy That Cholesterol and Saturated Fat Cause Heart Disease* (Washington, DC: NewTrends, 2000), 32–33.
13. *Nutrition Week*, March 22, 1991, 2–3.
14. Ravnskov, *The Cholesterol Myths*, 104.
15. E. Somer, "Minerals," in *The Essential Guide to Vitamins and Minerals* (New York: Harper Perennial, 1995), 89–94.
16. Sally Fallon and Mary Enig, *Eat Fat, Lose Fat* (New York: Hudson Street Press/Penguin, 2005), 51–52.
17. P. C. Elwood et al., "Milk Consumption, Stroke, and Heart Attack Risk: Evidence from the Caerphilly Cohort of Older Men," *Journal of Epidemiology and Community Health* 59 (2005): 502–5.
18. P. Reaven, S. Parthasarathy, B. J. Grasse, E. Miller, F. Almazan, F. H. Mattson, J. C. Khoo, D. Steinberg, and J. L. Witztum, "Feasibility of Using an Oleate-Rich Diet to Reduce the Susceptibility of Low-Density Lipoprotein to Oxidative

Modification in Humans," *American Journal of Clinical Nutrition* 54, no. 4 (1991): 701–6.

19. M. L. Kelly, E. S. Kolver, D. E. Bauman, M. E. Van Amburgh, and L. D. Muller, "Effect of Intake of Pasture on Concentrations of Conjugated Linoleic Acid in Milk of Lactating Cows," *Journal of Dairy Science* 81, no. 6 (1998): 1630–36. See also T. R. Dhiman, G. R. Anand, L. D. Satter, and M. W. Pariza, "Conjugated Linoleic Acid Content of Milk from Cows Fed Different Diets," *Journal of Dairy Science* 82, no. 10 (1999): 2146–56.
20. Laurie S. Z. Greenberg and Darcy Klasna, "The Marketing Potential of Conjugated Linoleic Acid (CLA) in Cheese: A Market Scan," Cooperative Development Services, May 2002, 9.
21. W. Campbell, M. A. Drake, and D. K. Larick, "The Impact of Fortification with Conjugated Linoleic Acid (CLA) on the Quality of Fluid Milk," *Journal of Dairy Science* 86 (2003): 48.
22. *California Morbidity Weekly Report*, March 31, 1989.
23. Martha M. Kramer, F. Latzke, and M. M. Shaw, "A Comparison of Raw, Pasteurized, Evaporated and Dried Milks as Sources of Calcium and Phosphorus for the Human Subject," *Journal of Biological Chemistry* 79 (1928): 283–95.
24. Madeleine Vedel, "Saving the Raw Milk Cheeses of Provençe," *Wise Traditions in Food, Farming and the Healing Arts* (newsletter of the Weston A. Price Foundation), 5, no. 4 (2004): 60–65.
25. X. Z. Ding et al., "Anti-Pancreatic Cancer Effects of Myristoleic Acid," *Pancreatology* 3 (2003): 209–69.
26. Schmid (*The Untold Story of Milk*) found the Mayo Clinic study. See also Bernarr Macfadden, *The Miracle of Milk: How to Use the Milk Diet Scientifically at Home* (Mcfadden Publications, 1924).
27. M. B. Zemel, "Role of Dietary Calcium and Dairy Products in Modulating Adiposity," *Lipids* 38, no. 2 (2003): 139–46.

3. *Real Meat*

1. Nichola Fletcher, "Hunting for Fat, Searching for Lean," in *The Fat of the Land: Proceedings of the Oxford Symposium on Food and Cookery, 2002*, ed. Harlan Walker (Bristol: Footwork, 2003), 88.
2. G. G. Khachatourians, "Agricultural Use of Antibiotics and the Evolution and Transfer of Antibiotic-Resistant Bacteria," *Canadian Medical Association Journal* 159, no. 9 (1998): 1129–36.
3. The figures refer to the period from June 1, 2004, to May 31, 2005.
4. Anne Dolamore, "Jack Sprat's Horror: Lardo Rediscovered," in *The Fat of the Land*, 76.
5. Bruce Kraig, "Fried in the Heartland," in *The Fat of the Land*, 169.
6. D. B. Mutetikka and D. C. Mahan, "Effect of Pasture, Confinement, and Diet

Fortification with Vitamin E and Selenium on Reproducing Gilts and Their Progeny," *Journal of Animal Science* 71 (1993): 3211.

7. C. H. Chiu, T. L. Wu, L. H. Su, C. Chu, J. H. Chia, A. J. Kuo, M. S. Chien, and T. Y. Lin, "The Emergence in Taiwan of Fluoroquinolone Resistance in *Salmonella enterica* Serotype Choleraesuis," *New England Journal of Medicine* 346, no. 6 (2002): 413–19.
8. Nicolette Hahn Niman, "The Unkindest Cut," *New York Times*, March 7, 2005.
9. A. A. Ojeniyi, "Public Health Aspects of Bacterial Drug Resistance in Modern Battery and Town/Village Poultry," *Acta Veterinaria Scandinavica* 30, no. 2 (1989): 127–32.
10. L. Horrigan, R. S. Lawrence, and P. Walker, "How Sustainable Agriculture Can Address the Environmental and Human Health Harms of Industrial Agriculture," *Environmental Health Perspectives* 110, no. 5 (2002): 445–56.
11. G. D. Bailey, B. A. Vanselow, M. A. Hornitzky, S. I. Hum, G. J. Eamens, P. A. Gill, K. H. Walker, and J. P. Cronin, "A Study of the Foodborne Pathogens: Campylobacter, Listeria and Yersinia, in Faeces from Slaughter-Age Cattle and Sheep in Australia," *Communicable Diseases Intelligence* 27, no. 2 (2003): 249–57.
12. T. R. Callaway, R. O. Elder, J. E. Keen, R. C. Anderson, and D. J. Nisbet, "Forage Feeding to Reduce Preharvest Escherichia coli Populations in Cattle, a Review," *Journal of Dairy Science* 86, no. 3 (2003): 852–60.
13. R. J. Nicolosi, E. J. Rogers, D. Kritchevsky, J. A. Scimeca, and P. J. Huth, "Dietary Conjugated Linoleic Acid Reduces Plasma Lipoproteins and Early Aortic Atherosclerosis in Hypercholesterolemic Hamsters," *Artery* 22, no. 5 (1997): 266–77.
14. Y. Park, K. J. Albright, W. Liu, J. M. Storkson, M. E. Cook, and M. W. Pariza, "Effect of Conjugated Linoleic Acid on Body Composition in Mice," *Lipids* 32, no. 8 (1997): 853–58. See also D. B. West, J. P. Delany, P. M. Camet, F. Blohm, A. A. Truett, and J. Scimeca, "Effects of Conjugated Linoleic Acid on Body Fat and Energy Metabolism in the Mouse," *American Journal of Physiology* 275, no. 3, pt. 2 (1998): R667–72.
15. P. Baghurst, S. Record, and J. Syrette, "Does Red Meat Cause Cancer?" *Australian Journal of Nutrition and Dietetics* 54 (1997): S1–44.
16. C. Ip, J. A. Scimeca, et al., "Conjugated Linoleic Acid. A Powerful Anticarcinogen from Animal Fat Sources," *Cancer* 74, no. 3 (1994): S1050–54.
17. C. Ip, S. F. Chin, J. A. Scimeca, and M. W. Pariza, "Mammary Cancer Prevention by Conjugated Dienoic Derivative of Linoleic Acid," *Cancer Research* 51, no. 22 (1991): 6118–24.
18. A. R. Eynard and C. B. Lopez, "Conjugated Linoleic Acid (CLA) Versus Saturated Fats/Cholesterol: Their Proportion in Fatty and Lean Meats May Affect the Risk of Developing Colon Cancer," *Lipids in Health and Disease* 2 (2003): 6.
19. A. Aro et al., "Inverse Association Between Dietary and Serum Conjugated Linoleic Acid and Risk of Breast Cancer in Postmenopausal Women," *Nutrition and Cancer* 38, no. 2 (2000): 151–57.

20. K. Sundram, K. C. Hayes, and O. H. Siru, "Dietary Palmitic Acid Results in Lower Serum Cholesterol Than Does a Lauric-Myristic Acid Combination in Normolipemic Humans," *American Journal of Clinical Nutrition* 59, no. 4 (1994): 841–46.
21. Nichola Fletcher, "Hunting for Fat, Searching for Lean," in *The Fat of the Land: Proceedings of the Oxford Symposium on Food and Cookery, 2002*, ed. Harlan Walker (Bristol: Footwork, 2003), 82.
22. Mary Enig, *Know Your Fats: The Complete Primer for Understanding the Nutrition of Fats, Oils, and Cholesterol* (Silver Spring, MD: Bethesda Press, 2000), 84.
23. C. Lai, D. M. Dunn, M. F. Miller, and B. C. Pence, "Non-Promoting Effects of Iron from Beef in the Rat Colon Carcinogenesis Model," *Cancer Letters* 112 (1997): 87–91.
24. G. Parnaud, G. Peiffer, S. Tache, and D. E. Corpet, "Effect of Meat (Beef, Chicken, and Bacon) on Rat Colon Carcinogenesis," *Nutrition and Cancer* 32 (1998): 165–73.
25. B. C. Pence, M. J. Butler, D. M. Dunn, M. F. Miller, C. Zhao, and M. Landers, "Non-promoting Effects of Lean Beef in the Rat Colon Carcinogenesis Model," *Carcinogenesis* 16 (1995): 1157–60.
26. P. Baghurst, S. Record, and J. Syrette, "Does Red Meat Cause Cancer?" *Australian Journal of Nutrition and Dietetics* 54 (1997): S1–44.
27. Ward Nicholson, www.beyondveg.com/cat/paleodiet/. Used by permission from Ward Nicholson, granted in May 2004.
28. M. D. Holmes, G. A. Colditz, D. J. Hunter, S. E. Hankinson, B. Rosner, F. E. Speizer, and W. C. Willett, "Meat, Fish and Egg Intake and Risk of Breast Cancer," *International Journal of Cancer* 104 (2003): 221–27.
29. IARC WHO Europe Against Cancer, European Commission, "European Prospective Investigation into Cancer and Nutrition (EPIC)," www.ism.uit.no/kk/e/EPIC percent20international.htm (accessed May 1, 2004).
30. A. R. Eynard and C. B. Lopez, "Conjugated Linoleic Acid (CLA) Versus Saturated Fats/Cholesterol: Their Proportion in Fatty and Lean Meats May Affect the Risk of Developing Colon Cancer," *Lipids in Health and Disease* 2 (2003): 6.
31. A. Navarro, M. P. Diaz, S. E. Munoz, M. J. Lantieri, and A. R. Eynard, "Characterization of Meat Consumption and Risk of Colorectal Cancer in Cordoba, Argentina," *Nutrition* 19 (2003): 7–10.
32. Heterocyclic amines and polycyclic aromatic hydrocarbons.
33. A. P. Simopoulos, "The Importance of the Ratio of Omega-6/Omega-3 Essential Fatty Acids," *Biomedicine and Pharmacotherapy* 56, no. 8 (2002): 365–79.

4. *Real Fish*

1. Talk by Michel Odent attended by the author, *Midwifery Today* conference, Philadelphia, March 18, 2004.

2. Ibid.
3. Living inland presents one other nutritional risk: iodine deficiency. The American Midwest is called the "goiter belt" because the thyroid needs iodine, found in unrefined sea salt and seafood.
4. Blaine Harden, "Tribe Fights Dams to Get Diet Back," *Washington Post,* January 30, 2005.
5. A. P. Simopoulos, "Omega-3 Fats in Health and Disease and in Growth and Development," *American Journal of Clinical Nutrition*, 54, no. 3 (1991): 451.
6. Andrew L. Stoll, *The Omega-3 Connection: The Ground-Breaking Anti-Depression and Diet Program* (New York: Fireside, 2001), 72.
7. Ibid., 74.
8. M. L. Burr, et al., "Effects of Changes in Fat, Fish, and Fiber Intakes on Death and Myocardial Reinfarction: Diet and Reinfarction Trial (DART)," *Lancet* 2, no. 8666 (1989): 757–61.
9. J. E. Kinsella. "Effects of Polyunsaturated Fatty Acids on Factors Related to Cardiovascular Disease," *American Journal of Cardiology* 60, no. 12 (1987): 23G–32G.
10. Simopoulos, "Omega-3 Fats in Health and Disease and in Growth and Development," 448.
11. Stoll, *The Omega-3 Connection*, 44–45.
12. Talk by Michel Odent attended by the author.
13. B. J. Stordy, "Long Chain Polyunsaturated Fatty Acids, Educational Achievement, and Behavior: A Review of New Research, 1998–2002," Stordy Jones Nutrition Consultants, Guildford, England.
14. G. Hornstra, "Essential Fatty Acids in Mothers and Their Neonates," *American Journal of Clinical Nutrition* 71 (May 2000): S1262–1269.
15. David Horrobin was a pioneer in the development of therapies based on the biochemistry of fats. He sparked a minor revolution in fat research and founded two pharmaceutical companies. He died in 2003.
16. Jerome Burn, "Why Fat on the Brain Can Drive You Insane," *Financial Times*, April 14–15, 2001.
17. Michel Odent, "Mercury Exposure During the Primal Period," *Journal of Prenatal and Perinatal Psychology and Health* 18, no. 3 (2004): 212–20.
18. "Study Finds Government Advisories on Fish Consumption and Mercury May Do More Harm Than Good," press release, Harvard School of Public Health, October 19, 2005. See also Eric Nagourney, "Public Health: Before Avoiding Fish, a Word to the Wise," *New York Times,* October 25, 2005.
19. For the full report, see www.consumerlab.com. Another source of mercury is amalgam dental fillings. Replace them if you can.

5. Real Fruit and Vegetables

1. Marilyn Sterling, "Anthocyanins," *Nutrition and Science News*, December 2001.
2. For more, see Andrew Kimbrell, ed., *Fatal Harvest: The Tragedy of Industrial Agriculture* (Sausalito, CA: Foundation for Deep Ecology by arrangement with Island Press).
3. Felicity Lawrence, *Not on the Label: What Really Goes into the Food on Your Plate* (London: Penguin, 2004), 29–31.
4. "Chemicals Evaluated for Carcinogenic Potential," Office of Pesticide Programs, U.S. Environmental Protection Agency, July 19, 2004.
5. Alyson E. Mitchell et al., "Comparison of the Total Phenolic and Ascorbic Acid Content of Freeze-Dried and Air-Dried Marionberry, Strawberry, and Corn Grown Using Conventional, Organic, and Sustainable Agricultural Practices," *Journal of Agricultural Food Chemistry* 51, no. 5 (2003): 1237–41.
6. Judith DeCava, "The Lee Philosophy, Part 2," *Health and Healing Wisdom* (journal of the Price-Pottenger Nutrition Foundation) 29, no. 1 (2005): 14–18.

6. Real Fats

1. B. V. Howard et al., "Low-Fat Dietary Pattern and Risk of Cardiovascular Disease. The Women's Health Initiative Randomized Controlled Dietary Modification Trial." *Journal of the American Medical Association* 295 (2006): 655–666; and R. L. Prentice et al., "Low-Fat Dietary Pattern and Risk of Invasive Breast Cancer. The Women's Health Initiative Randomized Controlled Dietary Modification Trial." *Journal of the American Medical Association* 295 (2006): 629–642.
2. B. N. Ames, "Dietary Carcinogens and Anticarcinogens. Oxygen Radicals and Degenerative Diseases," *Science* 221, no. 4617 (1983): 1256–64.
3. "Findings," *Harper's*, July 2005, 100.
4. M. L. Garg et al., *FASEB Journal* 2, no. 4 (1988): A852; and R. M. Oliart Ros et al., "Meeting Abstracts," *AOCS* PROCEEDINGS, May 1998, 7, Chicago, Illinois.
5. Bruce J. German and Cora J. Dillard, "Saturated Fats: What Dietary Intake?" *American Journal of Clinical Nutrition* 80, no. 3 (2004): 550–59.
6. Comments to the 2005 Dietary Guidelines Advisory Committee submitted by the Weston A. Price Foundation on January 16, 2004. See also L. D. Lawson and F. Kummerow, *Lipids* 14 (1979): 501–3; and M. L. Garg, *Lipids* 24, no. 4 (1989): 334–39.
7. Kilmer McCully, *The Homocysteine Revolution: A Bold New Approach to the Prevention of Heart Disease* (Los Angeles: Keats, 1997), 115.
8. Mary Enig, *Know Your Fats: The Complete Primer for Understanding the Nutrition of Fats, Oils, and Cholesterol* (Silver Spring, MD: Bethesda Press, 2002), 187.

9. Testimony of Mary Enig, FDA Hearing on Exploring the Connections Between Weight Management and Food Labels and Packaging, docket no. 2003N–0338, "Trans Fatty Acids in Nutrition Labeling," November 20, 2003.
10. K. C. Hayes, *Canadian Journal of Cardiology* 11 (1995): Suppl. G, 39–46. See also Ronald P. Mensink. "Effects of Stearic Acid on Plasma Lipid and Lipoproteins in Humans," *Lipids* 40 (2005): 1201–5.
11. International Food Information Council Review: "Sorting Out the Facts About Fat," July 1998, International Food Information Council, www.ific.org/publi cations/reviews/fatir.cfm.
12. German, and Dillard, "Saturated Fats," 553.
13. Ibid., 550–59.
14. M. Leosdottir et al., "Dietary Fat Intake and Early Mortality Patterns—Data from the Malmo Diet and Cancer Study," *Journal of Internal Medicine* 258 (2005): 153–65.
15. K. C. Hayes and P. Khosla, "Dietary Fat Thresholds and Cholesterolemia," *FASEB Journal* 6 (1992): 2600–2607.
16. K. Sundram, K. C. Hayes, and O. H. Siru, "Dietary Palmitic Acid Results in Lower Serum Cholesterol Than Does a Lauric-Myristic Acid Combination in Normolipemic Humans," *American Journal of Clinical Nutrition* 59, no. 4 (1994): 841–46.
17. R. W. Owen, A. Giacosa, W. E. Hull, R. Haubner, G. Wurtele, B. Spiegelhalder, and H. Bartsch, "Olive-Oil Consumption and Health: The Possible Role of Antioxidants," *Lancet Oncology* 1 (2000): 107–12.
18. A. K. Kiritsakis; contrib. by E. B. Lenart, W. C. Willet, and R. J. Hernandez, *Olive Oil: From the Tree to the Table.* (Trumbull, CT: Food and Nutrition Press, 1998), 15.
19. P. Knickerbocker, *Olive Oil: From Tree to Table* (San Francisco: Chronicle Books, 1997), 16.
20. Kiritsakis et al., *Olive Oil*, 191.
21. D. M. Colquhoun, B. J. Hicks, and A. W. Reed, "Phenolic Content of Olive Oil Is Reduced in Extraction and Refining: Analysis of Phenolic Content of Three Grades of Olive and Ten Seed Oils," *Asia Pacific Journal of Clinical Nutrition* 5 (1996): 105–7.
22. Owen et al., "Olive-Oil Consumption and Health," 107–12.
23. A. Trichopoulou, K. Katsouyanni, S. Stuver, L. Tzala, C. Gnardellis, E. Rimm, and D. Trichopoulos, "Consumption of Olive Oil and Specific Food Groups in Relation to Breast Cancer Risk in Greece," *Journal of the National Cancer Institute* 87, no. 2 (1995): 110–16.
24. M. Fito, M. I. Covas, R. M. Lamuela-Raventos, J. Vila, L. Torrents, C. de la Torre, and J. Marrugat. "Protective Effect of Olive Oil and Its Phenolic Compounds Against Low Density Lipoprotein Oxidation," *Lipids* 35, no. 6 (2000): 633–38.
25. Fran McCullough, *Good Fat* (New York: Scribner, 2003), 115.
26. Bruce Fife, *The Healing Miracles of Coconut Oil*, revised 3rd ed. (Colorado Springs, CO: HealthWise, 2003), 61, 101–2.
27. Mary Enig, "Health and Nutritional Benefits from Coconut Oil: An Important

Functional Food for the 21st Century," presented at the AVOC Lauric Oils Symposium, Ho Chi Min City, Vietnam, April 25, 1996.

28. C. Calabrese, S. Myer, S. Munson, P. Turet, and T. C. Birdsall, "A Cross-over Study of the Effect of a Single Oral Feeding of Medium Chain Triglyceride Oil vs. Canola Oil on Post-ingestion Plasma Triglyceride Levels in Healthy Men," *Alternative Medicine Review* 4, no. 1 (1999): 23–28.
29. M. P. St.-Onge and P. J. Jones, "Physiological Effects of Medium-Chain Triglycerides: Potential Agents in the Prevention of Obesity," *Journal of Nutrition* 132, no. 3 (2002): 329–32.
30. J. M. Stanhope, V. M. Sampson, and I. A. Prior, "The Tokelau Island Migrant Study: Serum Lipid Concentration in Two Environments," *Journal of Chronic Disease* 34, nos. 2–3 (1981): 45–55.
31. Enig, "Health and Nutritional Benefits from Coconut Oil."
32. N. Nosaka, M. Kasai, M. Nakamura, I. Takahashi, M. Itakura, H. Takeuchi, T. Aoyama, H. Tsuji, M. Okazaki, and K. Kondo, "Effects of Dietary Medium-Chain Triacylglycerols on Serum Lipoproteins and Biochemical Parameters in Healthy Men," *Bioscience, Biotechnology, and Biochemistry* 66, no. 8 (2002): 1713–18.
33. H. Kaunitz, "Medium Chain Triglycerides (MCT) in Aging and Arteriosclerosis," *Journal of Environmental Pathology, Toxicology and Oncology* 6, nos. 3–4 (1986): 115–21.
34. Sundram et al., "Dietary Palmitic Acid Results in Lower Serum Cholesterol," 841–46.
35. T. K. Ng, K. Hassan, J. B. Lim, M. S. Lye, and R. Ishak, "Nonhypercholesterolemic Effects of a Palm-Oil Diet in Malaysian Volunteers," *American Journal of Clinical Nutrition* 53, no. 4 (1991): S1015–20.
36. Enig, "Health and Nutritional Benefits from Coconut Oil."
37. N. de Roos, E. Schouten, and M. Katan, "Consumption of a Solid Fat Rich in Lauric Acid Results in a More Favorable Serum Lipid Profile in Healthy Men and Women Than Consumption of a Solid Fat Rich in Trans Fatty Acids," *Journal of Nutrition* 131, no. 2 (2001): 242–45.

7. *Industrial Fats*

1. A form of trans fats does occur naturally in ruminants, or grass eaters. It is the precursor to the omega-6 fatty acid conjugated linoleic acid, the anticancer agent found in the fat of grass-fed cattle. But this natural trans fat is chemically different from industrial trans fat and quite safe.

2. Linda Joyce Forristal, "The Rise and Fall of Crisco," www.motherlindas.com. The article first appeared in the Summer 2001 issue of *Wise Traditions*, the newsletter of the Weston A. Price Foundation.
3. Uffe Ravnskov, *The Cholesterol Myths: Exposing the Fallacy That Saturated*

Fat and Cholesterol Cause Heart Disease (Washington, DC: NewTrends, 2000), 229.

4. A. Ascherio, M. J. Stampfer, and W. C. Willett, "Trans Fatty Acids and Coronary Heart Disease," background and scientific review prepared by the Department of Nutrition and Epidemiology, Harvard School of Public Health; the Channing Laboratory, Department of Medicine, Brigham and Women's Hospital, November 15, 1999.
5. N. M. de Roos, M. L. Bots, and M. B. Katan, "Replacement of Dietary Saturated Fatty Acids by Trans Fatty Acids Lowers Serum HDL Cholesterol and Impairs Endothelial Function in Healthy Men and Women," *Arteriosclerosis, Thrombosis, and Vascular Biology* 21 (July 2001): 1233.
6. J. Booyens, C. C. Louwrens, and I. E. Katzeff, "The Role of Unnatural Dietary Trans and Cis Unsaturated Fatty Acids in the Epidemiology of Coronary Artery Disease," *Medical Hypotheses* 25, no. 3 (1988): 175–82.
7. J. T. Anderson, F. Grande, and A. Keys, "Hydrogenated Fats in the Diet and Lipids in the Serum of Man," *Journal of Nutrition* 75 (1961): 388–94.
8. Nina Teicholz, "Heart Breaker," *Gourmet*, June 2004.
9. Ascherio et al., "Trans Fatty Acids and Coronary Heart Disease."
10. Food and Nutrition Board, Institute of Medicine of the National Academies, National Academy of Sciences, "Letter Report on Dietary Reference Intakes for Trans Fatty Acids. Drawn from the Report on Dietary Reference Intakes for Energy, Carbohydrate, Fiber, Fat, Fatty Acids, Cholesterol, Protein, and Amino Acids," 2002, 4, 14.
11. www.bantransfats.com
12. The extraordinary advance of corn is well told in Michael Pollan, *The Omnivore's Dilemma: A Natural History of Four Meals* (2006); Richard Manning, *Against the Grain: How Agriculture Has Hijacked Civilization* (New York: Farrar, Straus and Giroux, 2004); and Margaret Visser, *Much Depends on Dinner: The Extraordinary History and Mythology, Allure and Obsessions, Perils and Taboos, of an Ordinary Meal* (New York: Grove Press, 1986).
13. A. P. Simopoulos, "Omega-3 Fats in Wild Plants, Nuts and Seeds," *Asia Pacific Journal of Clinical Nutrition* 11 (2002): S163–73.
14. M. Wardlaw Gordon, J. S. Hampl, and R. A. DiSilvestro, *Perspectives in Nutrition*, 6th ed. (New York: McGraw-Hill, 2004), 184–85.
15. Ibid., 185.
16. P. Reaven, S. Parthasarathy, B. J. Grasse, E. Miller, F. Almazan, F. H. Mattson, J. C. Khoo, D. Steinberg, and J. L. Witztum, "Feasibility of Using an Oleate-Rich Diet to Reduce the Susceptibility of Low-Density Lipoprotein to Oxidative Modification in Humans," *American Journal of Clinical Nutrition* 54, no. 4 (1991): 701–6.
17. Daniel Yam, Abraham Eliraz, and Elliot M. Berry, "Diet and Disease—the Israeli Paradox: Possible Dangers of a High Omega-6 Polyunsaturated Fatty Acid Diet," *Israeli Journal of Medical Science* 32, no. 11 (1996): 1134–43. See also more recent work by E. M. Berry and Gal Dubnov from the Department of Human Nutrition and Metabolism at Hadassah Medical School of Hebrew University in Jerusalem.

18. I highly recommend Jo Robinson's book, *Pasture Perfect: The Far-Reaching Benefits of Choosing Meat, Eggs, and Dairy Products from Grass-Fed Animals* (Vashon, WA: Vashon Island Press, 2004). Her Web site, www.eatwild.com, is frequently updated. There she writes, "If you were to inject a colony of rats with human cancer cells and then put some of the rats on a corn oil diet, some on a butterfat diet, and some on a beef fat diet, the ones given the omega-6 rich corn oil would be afflicted with larger and more aggressive tumors" (October 2005). Many studies back this up.
19. C. Calabrese, S. Myer, S. Munson, P. Turet, and T. C. Birdsall, "A Cross-over Study of the Effect of a Single Oral Feeding of Medium Chain Triglyceride Oil vs. Canola Oil on Post-ingestion Plasma Triglyceride Levels in Healthy Men," *Alternative Medicine Review* 4, no. 1 (1999): 23–28.

8. Other Real Foods

1. F. B. Hu, M. J. Stampfer et al., "A Prospective Study of Egg Consumption and Risk of Cardiovascular Disease in Men and Women," *Journal of the American Medical Association* 281, no. 15 (1999): 1387–94.
2. M. L. Slattery et al. "Carotenoids and Colon Cancer," *American Journal of Clinical Nutrition* 71 (2000): 575–82.
3. Felicity Lawrence, *Not on the Label: What Really Goes into the Food on Your Plate* (London: Penguin, 2004), 118.
4. See Susan Allport, *The Primal Feast: Food, Sex, Foraging and Love* (Lincoln, NE: iUniverse, 2003); Loren Cordain, *The Paleo Diet: Lose Weight and Get Healthy Eating the Food You Were Designed to Eat* (New York: John Wiley, 2002); and Richard Manning, *Against the Grain: How Agriculture Has Hijacked Civilization* (New York: Farrar, Straus and Giroux, 2004).
5. Commentary, "Consumption of High-Fructose Corn Syrup in Beverages May Play a Role in the Epidemic of Obesity," *American Journal of Clinical Nutrition* 79, no. 4 (2004): 537–43.
6. In *The Primal Feast,* Allport writes that one place where the rise of farming was not associated with declining health was the Nile Valley, where people fermented grain.
7. H. S. Qin ["A study on the effect of fermented soybean in preventing iron deficiency anemia in children"] *Zhonghua Yu Fang Yi Xue Za Zhi* 23, no. 6 (1989): 352–54 (article in Chinese).
8. I. E. Liener, "Implications of Antinutritional Components in Soybean Foods," *Critical Reviews in Food Science and Nutrition* 34, no. 1 (1994): 31–67; S. C. Sindhu and N. Khetarpaul, "Effect of Probiotic Fermentation on Antinutrients and In Vitro Protein and Starch Digestibilities of Indigenously Developed RWGT Food Mixture," *Nutrition Health* 16, no. 3 (2002): 173–81.
9. Liener, "Implications of Antinutritional Components in Soybean Foods."

10. A. P. Simopoulos, "The Importance of the Ratio of Omega-6/Omega-3 Essential Fatty Acids," *Biomedicine and Pharmacotherapy* 56, no. 8 (2002): 365–79.
11. *American Journal of Clinical Nutrition* 71, no. 5 (2000): 1166–69.
12. See, for example, these studies on soy and menopause: S. K. Quella, C. L. Loprinzi, D. L. Barton, J. A. Knost, J. A. Sloan, B. I. LaVasseur, D. Swan, K. R. Krupp, K. D. Miller, and P. J. Novotny, "Evaluation of Soy Phytoestrogens for the Treatment of Hot Flashes in Breast Cancer Survivors: A North Central Cancer Treatment Group Trial," *Journal of Clinical Oncology* 18, no. 5 (2000): 1068–74; D. C. Knight, J. B. Howes, J. A. Eden, L. G. Howes, "Effects on Menopausal Symptoms and Acceptability of Isoflavone-Containing Soy Powder Dietary Supplementation," *Climacteric* 4, no. 1 (2001): 13–18; C. L. Van Patten, I. A. Olivotto, G. K. Chambers, K. A. Gelmon, T. G. Hislop, E. Templeton, A. Wattie, and J. C. Prior, "Effect of Soy Phytoestrogens on Hot Flashes in Postmenopausal Women with Breast Cancer: A Randomized, Controlled Clinical Trial," *Journal of Clinical Oncology* 20, no. 6 (2002): 1449–55; and M. Penotti, E. Fabio, A. B. Modena, M. Rinaldi, U. Omodei, and P. Vigano, "Effect of Soy-Derived Isoflavones on Hot Flashes, Endometrial Thickness, and the Pulsatility Index of the Uterine and Cerebral Arteries, *Fertility and Sterility* 79, no. 5 (2003): 1112–17.
13. A. Cassidy, S. Bingham, and K. Setchell, "Biological Effects of a Diet of Soy Protein Rich in Isoflavones on the Menstrual Cycle of Premenopausal Women," *American Journal of Clinical Nutrition* 60, no. 3 (1994): 333–40.
14. See, for example, these studies on soy and breast cancer: D. F. McMichael-Phillips, C. Harding, M. Morton, S. A. Roberts, A. Howell, C. S. Potten, and N. J. Bundred, "Effects of Soy-Protein Supplementation on Epithelial Proliferation in the Histologically Normal Human Breast," *American Journal of Clinical Nutrition* 68, no. 6 (1998): S1431–35; N. L. Petrakis, S. Barnes, E. B. King, J. Lowenstein, J. Wiencke, M. M. Lee, R. Miike, M. Kirk, and L. Coward, "Stimulatory Influence of Soy Protein Isolate on Breast Secretion in Pre- and Postmenopausal Women," *Cancer Epidemiology Biomarkers and Prevention* 5, no. 10 (1996): 785–94; M. L. de Lemos, "Effects of Soy Phytoestrogens Genistein and Daidzein on Breast Cancer Growth," *Annals of Pharmacotherapy* 35, no. 9 (2001): 1118–21 (de Lemos found that *low* concentrations of soy phytoestrogens seem to promote the growth of breast tumors, while *high* concentrations appear to have a protective effect against breast tumor growth, so that "it is unclear whether tumor stimulation or inhibition would predominate in patients taking dietary soy supplements . . . Until long-term human studies are available, patients should be advised that the safety of taking large amounts of soy has not been established in this population and that other measures [e.g., lifestyle, diet, nonhormonal therapies] are available for controlling menopausal symptoms"); C. Y. Hsieh, R. C. Santell, S. Z. Haslam, and W. G. Helferich, "Estrogenic Effects of Genistein on the Growth of Estrogen Receptor-Positive Human Breast Cancer (MCF-7) Cells *In Vitro* and *In Vivo*," *Cancer Research* 58, no. 17 (1998); 3833–38; C. D. Allred, K. F. Allred, Y. H. Ju, S. M. Virant, and W. G. Helferich, "Soy Diets Containing Varying Amounts of Genistein Stimulate Growth of Estrogen-Dependent (MCF-7) Tumors in a Dose-Dependent Manner," *Cancer Research* 61, no. 13 (2001): 5045–50; and M. S. Kurzer,

"Phytoestrogen Supplement Use by Women," *Journal of Nutrition* 133, no. 6 (2003): S1983–86.

15. John W. Erdman et al., "Not All Soy Products Are Created Equal: Caution Needed in Interpretation of Research Results," *Journal of Nutrition* 134 (May 2004): S1229–33.
16. M. J. Messina and C. L. Loprinzi, "Soy for Breast Cancer Survivors: A Critical Review of the Literature," *Journal of Nutrition* 131, no. 11 (2001): S3095–3108.
17. They include William Helferich, professor of nutrition at the University of Illinois ("Soy Processing Influences Growth of Estrogen-Dependent Breast Cancer Tumors in Mice," *Carcinogenesis*, published online May 6, 2004 at www.uiuc.edu); the American Cancer Society; and Barry Sears, *The Soy Zone* (New York: HarperCollins, 2000).
18. Dr. Susan Love commented on the Helferich study in *Artemis*, a newsletter of the Breast Cancer Center at Johns Hopkins, June 2004.
19. Bradley J. Wilcox et al., *The Okinawa Program* (New York: Three Rivers Press, 2001), 114.
20. A. S. Sandberg, "Bioavailability of Minerals in Legumes," *British Journal of Nutrition* 88 (2002) Suppl. no. 3, 281–85.
21. A. M. Hutchins, J. L. Slavin, and J. W. Lampe, "Urinary Isoflavonoid Phytoestrogen and Lignan Excretion After Consumption of Fermented and Unfermented Soy Products," *Journal of the American Dietetic Association* 95, no. 5 (1995): 545–51.
22. The FDA specialists were D. M. Sheehan and D. R. Doerge. The letter included pages of citations supporting their view. (Dockets Management Branch [HFA-305], Food and Drug Administration, February 18, 1999.)
23. Y. Ishizuki, Y. Hirooka, Y. Murata, and K. Togashi, "The Effects on the Thyroid Gland of Soybeans Administered Experimentally in Healthy Subjects," *Nippon Naibunpi Gakkai Zasshi* 767, no. 5 (1991): 622–29.
24. Paper by Dr. Mike Fitzpatrick of New Zealand, "Soya Infant Formula: The Health Concerns," cited in Carol Simontacchi, *The Crazy Makers: How the Food Industry Is Destroying Our Brains and Harming Our Children* (New York: Jeremy Tarcher/Putnam, 2000), 75.
25. D. M. Sheehan, "Isoflavone Content of Breast Milk and Soy Formulas: Benefits and Risks" (letter), *Clinical Chemistry* 43, no. 5 (1997): 850–52.
26. Mary Enig and Sally Fallon, *Eat Fat, Lose Fat* (New York: Hudson Street Press, 2002), 97.
27. They include: the U.S. study MRFIT (analysis in 1997 and 1999), the Scottish Heart Health Study (1997), the National Health and Nutrition Examination Survey (1998), and a meta-analysis of many studies in the British Medical Journal (2002).
28. W. C. Hillel et al., "Sodium Intake and Mortality in the NHANES II Follow-Up Study," *American Journal of Medicine* 119 (2006): 275.e7–275.e14.
29. Davide Grassi, Cristina Lippi, Stefano Necozione, Giovambattista Desideri, and Claudio Ferri, "Short-Term Administration of Dark Chocolate Is Followed by a Significant Increase in Insulin Sensitivity and a Decrease in Blood Pressure in Healthy Persons," *American Journal of Clinical Nutrition.* 81 no. 3 (2005): 611–14.

9. *Beyond Cholesterol*

1. M. Muenke and M. M. Cohen Jr. "Genetic Approaches to Understanding Brain Development: Holoprosencephaly as a Model," *Mental Retardation and Developmental Disabilities Research Reviews* 6, no. 1 (2000): 15–21.
2. M. Wardlaw Gordon, J. S. Hampl, and R. A. DiSilvestro, *Perspectives in Nutrition*, 6th ed. (New York: McGraw-Hill, 2004), 194–96.
3. Anthony Colpo, "LDL Cholesterol: 'Bad' Cholesterol, or Bad Science?" *Journal of American Physicians and Surgeons* 10, no. 3 (2005), 83–89.
4. J. S. Garrow, W. P. T. James, and A. Ralph, *Human Nutrition and Dietetics*, 10th ed. (New York: Churchill Livingstone, 2002), 111.
5. "Fats and Cholesterol—the Good, the Bad, and the Healthy Diet," *The Nutrition Source: Knowledge and Information for Healthy Eating*, Harvard School of Public Health, June 16, 2003, available online at: www.hsph.harvard.edu/nutritionsource.
6. R. L. Duyff and the American Dietetic Association, *American Dietetic Association Complete Food and Nutrition Guide,* 2nd ed. (Hoboken, NJ: John Wiley, 2002), 65.
7. Enig, *Know Your Fats*, 57.
8. A. P. Simopoulos, "Omega-3 Fatty Acids in Health and Disease and in Growth and Development," *American Journal of Clinical Nutrition* 54, no. 3 (1991): 449.
9. See McCully and McCully, *The Heart Revolution*, 42–44.
10. Theodore B. Van Itallie, "Ancel Keys: A Tribute," *Nutrition and Metabolism*, February 14, 2005.
11. Mary Enig, "Health and Nutritional Benefits from Coconut Oil: An Important Functional Food for the 21st Century," presented at the AVOC Lauric Oils Symposium, Ho Chi Min City, Vietnam, April 25, 1996.
12. Ravnkov, *The Cholesterol Myths*, 16–17.
13. Stephen Phinney's letter about Keys appeared on www.nutritionandmetabolism.com on February 28, 2005. It was a response to Theodore B. Van Itallie, "Ancel Keys: A Tribute," in the February 14 issue of *Nutrition and Metabolism.*
14. Correspondence with the author, July 23, 2005.
15. These figures are from the American Heart Association. Statistics vary, and there are many different cardiovascular diseases. The Centers for Disease Control says heart disease killed 696,000 people in 2002 and strokes killed 162,000.
16. Centers for Disease Control, *Morbidity and Mortality Weekly Report* 48, no. 30 (1999): 649–56.
17. S. McCully, *The Homocysteine Revolution*, 58.
18. R. J. Havlik and M. Feinleib, "Proceedings of the Conference on the Decline in Coronary Heart Disease Mortality, October 24–25, 1978," NIH Publication no. 79–1610, May 1979.
19. "Cholesterol and Coronary Heart Disease: Screening and Treatment," *Effective Health Care* (National Health Service Centre for Reviews and Dissemination) 4, no. 1 (1998): 1.
20. See three studies: K. C. Hayes, *Canadian Journal of Cardiology* 11 (1995): Suppl.

G, 39–46; K. C. Hayes and P. Khosla, "Dietary Fatty Acid Thresholds and Cholesterolemia," *FASEB Journal* 6 (1992): 2600–2607; and K. Sundram, K. C. Hayes, and O. H. Siru, "Dietary Palmitic Acid Results in Lower Serum Cholesterol Than Does a Lauric-Myristic Acid Combination in Normolipemic Humans," *American Journal of Clinical Nutrition* 59, no. 4 (1994): 841–46.

21. *American Journal of Clinical Nutrition* 74 (December 2001): 730–36.
22. D. B. Shestov et al., "Increased Risk of Coronary Heart Disease Death in Men with Low Total and Low-Density Lipoprotein Cholesterol in the Russian Lipid Research Clinics Prevalence Follow-up Study," *Circulation* (journal of the American Heart Association) 88 (1993): 846–53.
23. Simopoulos, "Omega-3 Fats in Health and Disease and in Growth and Development," 458.
24. K. M. Anderson, W. P. Castelli, and D. Levy, "Cholesterol and Mortality. Thirty years of Follow-up from the Framingham Study," *Journal of the American Medical Association* 257, no. 16 (1987): 2176–80.
25. Enig, *Know Your Fats*, 78.
26. For current official guidelines, see the National Cholesterol Education Program at www.nhlbi.nih.gov/about/ncep. For a skeptical view, search for cholesterol at www.mercola.com.
27. Alex Berenson, "Lipitor or Generic? Billion-Dollar Battle Looms," *New York Times*, October 15, 2005.
28. N. Schupf et al., "Relationship Between Plasma Lipids and All-Cause Mortality in Non-Demented Elderly," *Journal of the American Geriatrics Society* 53 (2005): 219–229.
29. "OTC Statins: A Bad Decision for Public Health," editorial, *Lancet* 363, no. 9422 (2004).
30. International Coenzyme Q_{10} Association to U.S. Food and Drug Administration, September 5, 2001. The International Coenzyme Q_{10} Association, a body of scientists and medical professionals who conduct extensive research on coenzyme Q_{10}, issued a letter to the FDA, noting that statins block the biosynthesis of coenzyme Q_{10}. Ironically, coenzyme Q_{10} is critical for proper heart function, and the letter states that "although statin therapy has been shown to have benefits, the long-term response in ischemic heart disease may have been blunted due to the CoQ_{10} depleting effect" and cites several sources. See also Cordain, "Dietary Macronutrient Ratios and Their Effect on Biochemical Indicators of Risk for Heart Disease."
31. Talk by Peter Langsjoen, "CoQ_{10} Depletion: The Achilles" Heel of the Statin Crusade: A Review of Published Animal and Human Trials Showing Statin-Induced Coenzyme Q_{10} Depletion Resulting in Muscle Wasting and Heart Failure," Weston A. Price Foundation, annual conference, May 4, 2003, attended by the author. Langsjoen confirmed to the author that this was still his practice with heart patients in a talk on November 13, 2005 titled "The Clinical Implications of Statin-Induced Coenzyme Q_{10} Depletion" at the Weston A. Price Foundation Conference in Chantilly, Virginia. See also Peter Langsjoen, "Overview of the Use of CoQ_{10} in Cardiovascular Disease," *Biofactors* 9, nos. 2–3 (1999): 273–84.

32. Correspondence with the author, June 18, 2004. For more information from Barry Groves, see www.second-opinions.co.uk.
33. On June 21, 2004, Uffe Ravnskov provided the author with an English translation of a chapter titled "The Benefits of High Cholesterol" in the second German edition (2004) of *The Cholesterol Myths*. See also H. M. Krumholz, T. E. Seeman, S. S. Merrill, C. F. Mendes de Leon, V. Vaccarino, D. I. Silverman, R. Tsukahara, A. M. Ostfeld, and L. F. Berkman, "Lack of Association Between Cholesterol and Coronary Heart Disease Mortality and Morbidity and All-Cause Mortality in Persons Older than 70 Years," *Journal of the American Medical Association* 272, no. 17 (1994): 1335–40.
34. I. J. Schatz, K. Masaki, K. Yano, R. Chen, B. L. Rodriguez, and J. D. Curb, "Cholesterol and All-Cause Mortality in Elderly People from the Honolulu Heart Program: A Cohort Study," *Lancet* 358, no. 9279 (2001): 351–55.
35. O. Gatchev, L. Rastam, G. Lindberg, B. Gullberg, G. A. Eklund, and S. O. Isacsson, "Subarachnoid Hemorrhage, Cerebral Hemorrhage, and Serum Cholesterol Concentration in Men and Women," *Annals of Epidemiology* 3, no. 4 (1993): 403–9. See also D. R. Jacobs, "The Relationship Between Cholesterol and Stroke," *Health Rep* 6, no. 1 (1994): 87–93; and H. Iso, D. R. Jacobs Jr. D. Wentworth, J. D. Neaton, and J. D. Cohen, "Serum Cholesterol Levels and Six-Year Mortality from Stroke in 350,977 Men Screened for the Multiple Risk Factor Intervention Trial," *New England Journal of Medicine* 320, no. 14 (1989): 904–10.
36. *New England Journal of Medicine* 342 (2000): 836–43.
37. Scott Deron reports on the 2002 study in *C-Reactive Protein*. The 2005 study appeared in the *Journal of the American Medical Association* 294, no. 3 (2005).
38. David J. A. Jenkins et al., "Direct Comparison of Dietary Portfolio of Cholesterol-Lowering Foods with a Statin in Hypercholesterolemic Participants," *American Journal of Clinical Nutrition* 81, no. 2 (2005): 380–87.
39. Two of McCully's professors at Harvard were pioneers in the field of cholesterol metabolism. Louis K. Fieser was the Sheldon Emery Professor of Organic Chemistry at Harvard. He published the classic method for purification of cholesterol. He and several students and colleagues first fed oxidized cholesterol to rabbits to produce atherosclerotic plaques. Konrad E. Bloch was professor of chemistry at Harvard and winner of the Nobel Prize in Physiology or Medicine in 1964. He and Fyodor Lynen won the Nobel Prize for working out the biosynthesis of cholesterol.
40. Interview with the author, May 20, 2004, New York City.
41. P. Reaven, S. Parthasarathy, B. J. Grasse, E. Miller, F. Almazan, F. H. Mattson, J. C. Khoo, D. Steinberg, and J. L. Witztum, "Feasibility of Using an Oleate-Rich Diet to Reduce the Susceptibility of Low-Density Lipoprotein to Oxidative Modification in Humans," *American Journal of Clinical Nutrition* 54, no. 4 (1991): 701–6.

Glossary

alpha-linolenic acid (ALA)—A polyunsaturated omega-3 fat, one of the two essential fatty acids (the other is linoleic acid, or LA). ALA is required for the formation of other omega-3 fats, EPA, DPA, and DHA, which are essential to brain, visual, and hormone function. It's easier for the body to get EPA, DPA, and DHA from fish. Think of ALA as the land-based omega-3 fat. For vegetarians, key sources of ALA are flaxseed oil (60 percent), walnut oil (10 percent), and canola oil (10 to 15 percent).

alpha-lipoic acid—An antioxidant essential for metabolism found in grass-fed meat. Most antioxidants are either fat- or water-soluble, but alpha-lipoic acid is both. It extends the life of other antioxidants, such as vitamins C and E, lowers blood sugar, and improves sensitivity to insulin.

antioxidants—Compounds that counter the effects of free radicals and prevent or delay undesirable oxidation, or damage by oxygen. Vitamin C is a water-soluble antioxidant, vitamin E a fat-soluble one, and alpha-lipoic acid is both water- and fat-soluble. Coenzyme Q_{10}, which is depleted by statins, is an antioxidant found in organ meats (especially heart), red meat, and fish. Sesame and olive oil are rich in antioxidants. Plants contain dozens of antioxidant compounds, including carotenoids. Antioxidants last mere hours in the body; that's why it's sensible to eat fresh, brightly colored fruit, berries, and vegetables every day.

arrhythmia—Irregular heartbeat. Sometimes follows a myocardial infarction, or heart attack. Omega-3 fats reduce the rate of fatal arrhythmia by 30 percent.

arteriosclerosis—A common condition in which the smooth, elastic walls of the artery (never veins) become stiff, possibly as a protective measure to keep the high arterial blood pressure from straining the walls. Increases with age.

atherogenesis—The formation of plaques, or atheromas, in the arterial wall.

atheroma (*plaque*)—Raised swollen areas in the arterial wall. Atheromas may burst, resulting in a blood clot and a heart attack (in a coronary artery) or stroke (in an artery leading to the brain). Atheromas contain fats, cholesterol, white blood cells, and calcium.

atherosclerosis—Multiple atheromas. Atherosclerosis is more pronounced in people with high blood pressure and worsens with age. When an artery is obstructed, heart disease can result. However, many people who die of heart disease do not have atherosclerosis; something else blocks the blood flow.

betaine—A vitaminlike nutrient found in eggs, liver, and beets. Betaine reduces homocysteine and thus helps prevent heart disease.

bile acid—Manufactured in the liver from cholesterol and stored in the gallbladder, bile acid is essential for the emulsification and digestion of fats.

canola oil—The mostly monounsaturated oil from rapeseed, a plant in the genus *Brassica*, which includes broccoli and cabbage. Originally rapeseed was high in erucic acid, a toxic monounsaturated fat, but modern hybrids developed in Canada are low in erucic acid. Canola oil is frequently refined and partially hydrogenated in processed foods.

cardiovascular diseases—Diseases of the heart and vascular system, including heart disease, high blood pressure, congestive heart failure, stroke, and others.

carotenoids—Antioxidant plant pigments that are mainly fat-soluble. Examples: beta-carotene (sweet potato, carrot, kale, mango), lutein (melon, guava, spinach, collards), lycopene (tomatoes), and zeaxanthin (corn, nectarines, oranges, papaya). Eating carotenoids helps prevent cardiovascular diseases and cancer. Lutein and zeaxanthin, also found in egg yolks, may prevent the eye disease macular degeneration.

cholesterol—A molecule, chemically a sterol, made chiefly in the liver. It forms all cell membranes and makes up most of brain and nervous tissue. Cholesterol is required for production of bile acids, vitamin D, and the sex hormones (estrogens and androgens). It's a repair agent, rushing to the scene when arterial walls are damaged. Cholesterol is carried in the blood by the lipoproteins HDL and LDL. Cholesterol is found only in animal foods.

choline—A B–vitamin-like nutrient that is part of lecithin, which is found in egg yolks and butter. Choline is essential in the metabolism of fat and to the developing brain of the fetus. It reduces homocysteine and thus helps prevent heart disease.

coenzyme Q_{10} (CoQ_{10})—An antioxidant found in organ meats (especially heart), red meat, and fish. Statin drugs deplete CoQ_{10}, which is essential for heart function. Low CoQ_{10} is a risk factor for heart disease.

conjugated linoleic acid (CLA)—An omega-6 fat found in the fat of ruminant (grass-eating) animals. Grass-fed beef fat and butter are all but unique sources of CLA, an anticancer agent that also aids weight loss and builds lean muscle tissue. CLA is an unusual omega-6 fat in that it behaves like an omega-3 fat.

coronary heart disease (CHD)—See heart disease

C-reactive protein (CRP)—A protein made by the liver during acute inflammation. High CRP is a risk factor for heart disease.

docosahexaenoic acid (DHA)—An omega-3 fat essential to cell membranes, especially brain, eye, and sperm cells. Half the fat in the brain is DHA. Found chiefly in fish, DHA is used to form EPA. DHA can be manufactured in the body from alpha-linolenic acid (ALA), an essential fatty acid, but fish is the best source.

diabetes—A metabolic disease in which insulin does not work properly and sugar accumulates in the blood. In type 1 diabetes, the pancreas does not produce insulin. In type 2 diabetes (90 percent of cases), muscle cells are deaf to insulin, or "insulin-resistant." Obesity, sugar, excess of polyunsaturated vegetable oils, and a lack of omega-3 fats cause type 2. Prediabetes is called metabolic syndrome. Diabetes is a risk factor for heart disease.

eicosanoid—Several kinds of hormonelike agents, including prostaglandins, derived from the essential fatty acids. Omega-3 fats produce anti-inflammatory and calming eicosanoids, and omega-6 fats make inflammatory and reactive eicosanoids. The body needs both, but the industrial diet contains an excess of omega-6 fats and too few omega-3 fats, which leads to inflammation, diabetes, obesity, and heart disease.

emulsifier—An agent able to mix water and fat because it contains both water- and fat-soluble elements. The lecithin in egg yolks emulsifies mayonnaise. Bile acids emulsify fats in digestion.

eicosapentaenoic acid (EPA)—An omega-3 fat found chiefly in fish. EPA is required for the formation of eicosanoids, powerful hormonelike agents that control all cellular activity. EPA can be manufactured in the body from alpha-linolenic acid (ALA), an essential fatty acid.

epidemiology—The study of population and disease. Researchers look for risk factors and causes of disease.

essential fatty acids (EFA)—The omega-3 and omega-6 fats. They cannot be made by the body; hence they are "essential" and must be obtained through diet. From EFA, the body forms hormonelike agents called eicosanoids. EFA are essential to growth and brain and vision. If you don't eat enough EFA, the body will plunder its own stores. EFA deficiency is progressive and cumulative over generations. Pregnant and nursing women need large amounts of omega-3 fats to feed the baby's brain and prevent post-natal depression.

fat—A collection of triglycerides that are usually solid or semi-solid at room temperature.

fatty acid—An organic molecule made up of a chain of carbon atoms. Classified by the number of carbons (short-, medium-, long-, and very-long-chain fatty acids) and by whether the carbon atoms are saturated with hydrogen atoms (saturated or unsaturated). Fatty acids include oleic acid (in lard and olive oil), stearic acid (beef and chocolate), and lauric acid (coconut oil and breast milk).

flavonoids—Antioxidant compounds found in plants, especially brightly colored ones, such as sweet potatoes, cherries, and chocolate. Flavonoids fight cardiovascular diseases and cancer.

folic acid—An essential nutrient found in liver, eggs, green leafy vegetables, oysters, salmon, and beef. Prenatal deficiency of folic acid causes spina bifida in babies. Lack of folic acid elevates homocysteine, which causes heart disease.

free radicals—By-products of cell metabolism formed when oxygen is metabolized or burned. They damage cells and contribute to aging, cardiovascular diseases, and cancer. Antioxidants counter the effects of free radicals.

Gamma-linolenic acid (GLA)—A polyunsaturated omega-6 fatty acid found in the oils of borage, black currant seed, evening primrose, and Siberian pine nuts. The body can also make

GLA from the EFA linoleic acid (LA). GLA is an unusual omega-6 fat in that it tends to behave like an omega-3 fat. Eicosanoids derived from GLA reduce inflammation, dilate blood vessels, and reduce clotting. GLA also aids fat metabolism and treats premenstrual symptoms.

heart disease—The first stage of heart disease, angina, is restriction of blood to the heart. When the blood flow is stopped for a long time or stops totally, a heart attack (myocardial infarction) results. Together, angina and heart attack are heart disease. Heart disease is one of several cardiovascular diseases.

high-density lipoprotein (HDL)—Carries cholesterol from the bloodstream to the liver.

homocysteine—An amino acid that causes atherosclerosis. Lack of folic acid and vitamins B_6 and B_{12} elevates homocysteine.

hydrogenation—A chemical process that adds hydrogen to unsaturated double bonds in fats. Hydrogenation turns unsaturated, liquid oils into saturated, solid fats (such as corn oil into margarine) and creates unhealthy trans fats. Many processed foods contain hydrogenated and partially hydrogenated vegetable oils, which cause heart disease.

hypercholesterolemia—A rare genetic condition affecting about 1 percent of the population. The main symptom is high LDL. Hypercholesterolemics do not respond to changes in dietary cholesterol or saturated fats and often get atherosclerosis and heart disease early in life.

inflammation—The body's normal chemical response to injury or danger. White blood cells, platelets, and other healing agents rush to the injury, causing redness, swelling, warmth, and pain. Chronic inflammation (due to genetics, diet, infection, or some other cause) contributes to heart disease. Omega-6 fats in polyunsaturated vegetable oils lead to inflammation, while omega-3 fats prevent it. Inflammatory diseases resulting from lack of omega-3 fats include Crohn's, lupus, rheumatoid arthritis, and asthma. Fat cells promote inflammation, which may explain why being fat is a risk factor for heart disease.

insulin—A hormone produced by the pancreas and released when blood sugar rises after eating. Insulin directs the muscles to take sugar from the blood to muscles for use as immediate or short-term energy. When the muscles are deaf to insulin—"insulin resistant"—normal metabolism fails, and sugar (toxic in excess) accumulates in the blood. Excess sugar is stored as fat. Diabetes is a disease of insulin resistance.

isoflavones—Phytoestrogens, found in plants, which act like estrogens in the body. Isoflavones in soy foods may contribute to estrogen-dependent breast cancers.

lauric acid—A medium-chain saturated fat found in tropical oils such as coconut and palm and breast milk. Butter contains minor amounts (about 3 percent). A potent antimicrobial agent, it also stimulates metabolism and aids weight loss. Because lauric acid is stable (not easily damaged) at high temperatures, coconut oil is ideal for baking.

lecithin—An emulsifier in egg yolks and butter. Necessary for the proper digestion of cholesterol and fats.

linoleic acid (LA)—A polyunsaturated omega-6 fat in walnuts and flaxseed and one of the two essential fatty acids (the other is alpha-linolenic acid or ALA). LA is required for the formation of eicosanoids, hormonelike agents. Seed oils such as safflower (78 percent), sunflower (68 percent), and corn oil (57 percent) are rich in LA. The typical American diet contains far too much LA, which leads to obesity, diabetes, heart disease, cancer, and depression.

lipids—Fatty molecules including fats and oils. Lipids include fatty acids (such as oleic acid in lard and olive oil) and phospholipids (such as lecithin).

lipoprotein—A molecule that's part protein, part fat. It circulates in the blood, carrying cholesterol, homocysteine, and triglycerides.

lipoprotein (a) (Lp (a))—A unique lipoprotein that causes atherosclerosis and promotes clots. Trans fats raise Lp (a), and saturated fats lower it.

low-density lipoprotein (LDL)—Carries cholesterol from the liver to the blood. Oxidized LDL causes atherosclerosis.

metabolic syndrome—Also insulin resistance. Refers to several conditions involving chronically elevated insulin, including: belly fat, high blood pressure, low HDL, high LDL, and high triglycerides. Another sign of metabolic syndrome is normal cholesterol and high CRP—a sign of inflammation. First identified in 1989, metabolic syndrome is an early stage of diabetes, which is a predictor of kidney failure, stroke, and heart disease.

monounsaturated fats—Fatty acids with one double or unsaturated bond in the carbon chain such as oleic acid in olive oil, chicken fat, and lard. Monounsaturated fats are relatively stable and suitable for cooking, especially combined with saturated fats.

myocardial infarction (MI)—A heart attack. Occurs when a coronary artery supplying oxygen-rich blood to the heart muscle is blocked. If the heart is deprived of oxygen for more than a few minutes, heart cells die. Arrythmia, a chaotic heartbeat, may also occur.

oil—A collection of triglycerides that are usually liquid at room temperature.

omega-3 fats—Essential fatty acids that the body cannot make and must be obtained in the diet. ALA (in flaxseed, walnuts, purslane) and EPA and DHA (fish oils) are omega-3 fats. The omega family is essential for making eicosanoids. The industrial diet lacks omega-3 fats, which leads to obesity, diabetes, heart disease, cancer, and depression.

omega-6 fats—Essential fatty acids that the body cannot make and must be obtained in the diet. LA, gamma-linolenic acid, and arachidonic acid are omega-6 fats. The omega family is essential for making eicosanoids. The industrial diet contains too many omega-6 fats, which leads to obesity, diabetes, heart disease, cancer, and depression.

plaque—See atheroma

polyunsaturated fats—Fatty acids with two or more double or unsaturated bonds in the carbon chain. Most vegetable oils (corn, safflower, sunflower oil) are polyunsaturated and liquid at room temperature. Polyunsaturated fats are highly unstable and subject to oxidation, or damage, from heat and light. Fish oil is also polyunsaturated.

prostaglandins—Potent hormonelike agents, produced from the essential omega-3 and omega-6 fats and found in many body tissues. Prostaglandins are involved in all cellular activity. They affect inflammation, blood pressure, and metabolism, among many other bodily functions.

risk factor—A factor statistically associated with a disease. A risk factor may or may not *cause* disease. A risk factor that isn't causal is called a marker. Several hundred risk factors for heart disease include high homocysteine and CRP, inflammation, smoking, diabetes, gum disease, high blood pressure, and being overweight, sedentary, or male.

saturated fats—Fatty acids abundant in meat, lard, dairy foods, breast milk, and coconut oil. Saturated fats are usually solid at room temperature and stable at high temperatures, which makes them ideal for cooking and baking. Their carbon atoms are saturated with hydrogen atoms.

statins—Drugs used to block cholesterol synthesis. Stains deplete the body of the antioxidant CoQ_{10}, interfere with metabolism of EFA, damage the liver, and cause muscle weakness and memory loss.

thermic effect—The energy used to digest food. Protein has a higher thermic effect than carbohydrate or fat. Medium-chain saturated fats such as lauric acid (found in coconut oil) speed up metabolism compared with long-chain polyunsaturated fats such as those in corn oil.

thrombosis—A blood clot. Burst clots are one cause of heart attacks. Omega-3 fats reduce clotting.

trans fat—Produced when unsaturated fats undergo hydrogenation in which liquid oils (typically corn or soybean) are bombarded with hydrogen atoms to fill their unsaturated bonds to make them solid and shelf-stable. Trans fats cause heart disease, diabetes, cancer, arthritis, and other problems. A natural form of trans fat occurs in ruminants. A precursor to CLA, it is chemically different from synthetic trans fat and perfectly safe.

triglycerides—Three fatty acid molecules attached to a glycerol molecule. All fats and oils (lipids) are made of triglycerides.

unsaturated fats—Fatty acids with one or more double (carbon-to-carbon) bonds. A fatty acid with a single double bond is called monounsaturated; with two or more, it is polyunsaturated. Most vegetable oils are predominantly unsaturated.

vitamins—Discovered mostly between 1900 to 1930, the thirteen known vitamins are organic molecules essential in small amounts for health. They are either fat- or water-soluble.

Bibliography

Agatston, Arthur. *The South Beach Diet: The Delicious, Doctor-Designed, Foolproof Plan for Fast and Healthy Weight Loss.* New York: Random House, 2003.

Allport, Susan. *The Primal Feast: Food, Sex, Foraging, and Love.* Lincoln, NE: iUniverse, 2003. (Originally published by Harmony Books.)

Ashton, John, and Suzy Ashton. *A Chocolate a Day Keeps the Doctor Away.* New York: St. Martin's Press, 2003.

Atkins, Robert C. *Dr. Atkins Health Revolution: How Complementary Medicine Can Extend Your Life.* Boston: Bantam Books, 1989.

———. *Dr. Atkins New Diet Revolution.* New York: Avon Books/HarperCollins, 2002.

Audette, Ray. *Neanderthin: Eat Like a Caveman to Achieve a Lean, Strong, Healthy Body.* New York: St. Martin's Press, 1999.

Byrnes, Stephen. *Diet and Heart Disease: It's Not What You Think.* Warsaw, IN: Wendell W. Whitman, 2001.

Cordain, Loren. *The Paleo Diet: Lose Weight and Get Healthy Eating the Food You Were Designed to Eat.* New York: John Wiley, 2002.

Davis, Adelle. *Let's Eat Right to Keep Fit.* New York: Harcourt Brace Jovanovich, 1970.

———. *Let's Get Well.* New York: Harcourt Brace Jovanovich, 1965.

———. *Let's Have Healthy Children.* New York: Harcourt Brace Jovanovich, 1972.

de Langre, Jacques. *Seasalt's Hidden Powers.* Asheville, NC: Happiness Press, 1994.

Deron, Scott J. *C-Reactive Protein: Everything You Need to Know About CRP and Why It's More Important Than Cholesterol to Your Health.* New York: McGraw-Hill, 2004.

DesMaisons, Kathleen. *Potatoes Not Prozac: A Natural Seven-Step Dietary Plan to Control Your Cravings and Lose Weight, Recognize How Foods Affect the Way You Feel, and Stabilize the Level of Sugar in Your Blood.* New York: Fireside, 1999.

Diamond, Jared. *Guns, Germs, and Steel: The Fates of Human Societies.* New York: W. W. Norton, 1999.

Enig, Mary. *Know Your Fats: The Complete Primer for Understanding the Nutrition of Fats, Oils, and Cholesterol.* Silver Spring, MD: Bethesda Press, 2000.

Enig, Mary, and Sally Fallon. *Eat Fat, Lose Fat.* New York: Hudson Street Press, 2005.

Fallon, Sally, and Mary Enig. *Nourishing Traditions.* Revised 2nd ed. Washington, DC: NewTrends, 2001.

Fife, Bruce. *The Healing Miracles of Coconut Oil.* Revised 3rd ed. Colorado Springs, CO: HealthWise, 2003.

Garrow, J. S., W. P. T. James, and A. Ralph. *Human Nutrition and Dietetics.* 10th ed. New York: Churchill Livingstone, 2002.

Giles, Fiona. *Fresh Milk: The Secret Life of Breasts.* New York: Simon and Schuster, 2003.

Gittelman, Ann Louise. *Eat Fat, Lose Weight: How the Right Fats Can Make You Thin.* Lincolnwood, IL: Keats, 1999.

Graveline, Duane. *Lipitor: Thief of Memory.* Haverford, PA: Infinity, 2004.

Grohman, Joann S. *Keeping a Family Cow*. Dixfield, ME: Coburn Press, 2001.

———. *Real Food: Happy Choices for Hard Times*. Dixfield, ME: Coburn Press, 1995.

Gruberg, Edward R., and Stephen A. Raymond. *Beyond Cholesterol: Vitamin B_6, Arteriosclerosis, and Your Heart*. New York: St. Martin's Press, 1981.

Kauffman, Joel M. *Malignant Medical Myths*. West Conshohocken, PA: Infinity Publishing.

Kimbrell, Andrew, ed. *Fatal Harvest: The Tragedy of Industrial Agriculture*. Sausolito, CA: Foundation for Deep Ecology by arrangement with Island Press, 2002.

Kjaergaard, Thorkild. *The Danish Revolution, 1500–1800: An Ecohistorical Interpretation*. Cambridge: Cambridge University Press, 1994.

Krasner, D. *The Flavors of Olive Oil: A Tasting Guide and Cookbook*. New York: Simon and Schuster, 2002.

Lawrence, Felicity. *Not on the Label: What Really Goes into the Food on Your Plate*. London: Penguin, 2004.

Macfadden, Bernarr. *The Miracle of Milk: How to Use the Milk Diet Scientifically at Home*. Mcfadden Publications, 1924.

Mallet, Gina. *Last Chance to Eat: The Fate of Taste in a Fast Food World*. New York: W. W. Norton, 2004.

Manning, Richard. *Against the Grain: How Agriculture Has Hijacked Civilization*. New York: Farrar, Straus and Giroux, 2004.

McCullough, Fran. *Good Fat*. New York: Scribner, 2003.

McCully, Kilmer S. *The Homocysteine Revolution: Medicine for the New Millennium*. Los Angeles: Keats, 1997.

McCully, Kilmer S., and Martha McCully. *The Heart Revolution: The Extraordinary Discovery That Finally Laid the Cholesterol*

Myth to Rest and Put Good Food Back on the Table. New York: HarperPerennial, 1999.

McGee, Harold. *On Food and Cooking: The Science and Lore of the Kitchen*. New York: Fireside, 1997, and the revised edition, 2004.

Meggs, William Joe, and Carol Svec. *The Inflammation Cure: How to Combat the Hidden Factor Behind Heart Disease, Arthritis, Asthma, Diabetes, Alzheimer's Disease, Osteoporosis, and Other Diseases of Ageing*. New York: McGraw-Hill, 2004.

Montgomery, M. R. *A Cow's Life: The Surprising History of Cattle and How the Black Angus Came to Be Home on the Range*. New York: Walker, 2004.

Morgan, Elaine. *The Descent of Woman*. New York: Stein and Day, 1972.

Packer, Lester, and Carol Colman. *The Antioxidant Miracle*. New York: John Wiley, 1999.

Pinker, Steven. *The Language Instinct: The New Science of Language and the Mind*. London: Penguin, 1994.

Pottenger, Francis M., Jr. *Pottenger's Cats: A Study in Nutrition*. 2nd ed. La Mesa, CA: Price-Pottenger Nutrition Foundation, 1995.

Price, Weston A. *Nutrition and Physical Degeneration*. 6th ed. La Mesa, CA: Price-Pottenger Nutrition Foundation, 2000. (Originally published in 1939.)

Proulx, Annie, and Lew Nichols. *The Complete Dairy Foods Cookbook*. Emmaus, PA: Rodale Press, 1982.

Rath, Sara. *About Cows*. Stillwater, MN: Voyageur Press, 2000.

Ravnskov, Uffe. *The Cholesterol Myths: Exposing the Fallacy That Cholesterol and Saturated Fat Cause Heart Disease*. Washington, DC: NewTrends, 2000.

Robinson, Jo. *Pasture Perfect: The Far-Reaching Benefits of Choosing Meat, Eggs, and Dairy Products from Grass-Fed*

Animals. (Originally published as *Why Grass Is Best*.) Vashon, WA: Vashon Island Press, 2004.

Schmid, Ronald F. *Traditional Foods Are Your Best Medicine: Improving Health and Longevity with Native Nutrition*. Rochester, VT: Healing Press, 1997.

———. *The Untold Story of Milk: Green Pastures, Contented Cows and Raw Dairy Foods*. Washington, DC: NewTrends, 2003.

Schwarzbein, Diana, and Nancy Deville. *The Schwarzbein Principle: The Truth About Losing Weight, Being Healthy and Feeling Younger*. Deerfield Beach, FL: Health Communications, 1999.

Sears, Barry. *The Soy Zone*. New York: HarperCollins, 2000.

Shilhavy, Brian, and Marianita Jader Shilhavy. *Virgin Coconut Oil*. West Bend, WI: Tropical Traditions, 2004.

Sinatra, Stephen T. *The Coenzyme* Q_{10} *Phenomenon*. Lincolnwood, IL: Keats, 1998.

Snell, K. D. M. *Annals of the Labouring Poor: Social Change and Agrarian England, 1660 to 1900*. Cambridge: Cambridge University Press, 1985.

Stoll, Andrew. *The Omega-3 Connection: The Ground-Breaking Anti-Depression and Diet Program*. New York: Fireside, 2001.

Visser, Margaret. *Much Depends on Dinner: The Extraordinary History and Mythology, Allure and Obsessions, Perils and Taboos, of an Ordinary Meal*. New York: Grove Press, 1986.

Voisin, André. *Soil, Grass and Cancer: The Link Between Human and Animal Health and the Mineral Balance of the Soil*. Austin, TX: Acres U.S.A., 1999. (Originally published in 1959.)

Walker, Harlan, ed. *The Fat of the Land: Proceedings of the Oxford Symposium on Food and Cookery, 2002*. Bristol, England: Footwork, 2003.

Wardlaw, G. M., J. S. Hampl, and R. A. DiSilvestro. *Perspectives in Nutrition*. 6th ed. New York: McGraw-Hill, 2004.

Wilcox, Bradley J., et al. *The Okinawa Program*. New York: Three Rivers Press, 2001.

Wiley, T. S. *Lights Outs: Sleep, Sugar, and Survival*. New York: Pocket Books/Simon and Schuster, 2003.

Appreciation

I am grateful to my agent, Jennifer Unter, who worked hard to make this book possible and to make it a better one; to Cindy Embleton for her indispensable research; to grass farmers Joann Rogers and Joel Salatin for answering many questions; and to Kathy Belden at Bloomsbury for her astute suggestions. I am deeply thankful to Rob Kaufelt, Stephen Hargrave, Robin Shuster, and my wonderful family—Charles, Denise, and my parents—for many hours spent listening, reading, and editing. I could not have done it without you.

Index

A NOTE ON THE AUTHOR

Nina Planck grew up on a vegetable farm in Virginia. She was a speechwriter to the U.S. ambassador to Britain when she opened the first farmers' market in London on June 6, 1999. Six months later, she quit her job to open ten more markets, write *The Farmers' Market Cookbook*, and host a British television series on local food. In 2003, Nina created the Mount Pleasant Local Food Market in Washington, D.C. In New York City, she ran Greenmarket, the largest network of farmers' markets in the United States. Nina's new company, Real Food, runs markets for farmers and purveyors of regional and traditional foods.

www.RealFood.info
www.NinaPlanck.com